The
HEALTH
Address Book

A Directory of Health Support Groups

Third Edition

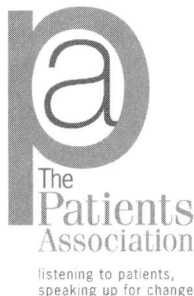

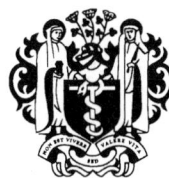

The
Patients
Association

listening to patients,
speaking up for change

The ROYAL
SOCIETY *of*
MEDICINE
PRESS *Limited*

THE HEALTH ADDRESS BOOK 3rd Edition

A Directory of Health Support Groups

Published by Royal Society of Medicine Press Ltd in collaboration with The Patients Association

Royal Society of Medicine Press Ltd
1 Wimpole Street, London W1G 0AE, UK
207 Westminster Road, Lake Forest, IL 60045, USA
www.rsmpress.co.uk

First published 1990
Second edition 1997
Third edition 2001

A catalogue record for this book is available from the British Library

ISBN 1-85315-455-5

© Royal Society of Medicine Press Ltd

Publisher: Peter Richardson

Project Manager: Nora Naughton

Phototypeset by Phoenix Photosetting, Chatham, Kent

Printed in Great Britain by Bell and Bain Ltd, Glasgow

Publishers Statement

The Patients Association and Royal Society of Medicine cannot accept responsibility for statements made in the directory section. The entries are based on information supplied or checked by the organisations concerned, edited where necessary to standardise presentation. While every effort has been made to ensure that details are accurate and up-to-date, some changes may have occurred between going to press and publication.

The Patients Association

The Patients Association aims to:

- Listen to patients and encourage people to tell their stories and relate their experiences of healthcare to us through our Patient-line, our Patients Voices magazine, and by individual personal contact

- Advise patients through our fact sheets, good practice material and self-help guides;

- Speak up for patients and, on the basis of what they tell us, support patients in speaking up for themselves to government, politicians, the Department of Health, health professionals, managers and industry;

- Campaign for improved health services from the patients' point of view, and for the development of a consumer-led health system in which patients are encouraged and enabled to make their own informed choices

President: Claire Rayner
Chairman: Vanessa Bourne
Director: Mike Stone

Criteria for Inclusion

The organisations listed in this directory are primarily voluntary organisations – that is, self-governing groups of people who have joined together voluntarily to take action for the betterment of the community. Organisations affiliated to any political party are not included, nor are organisations set up primarily for financial gain. The inclusion of any entry describing an organisation and its activities should not be taken to mean that The Patients Association or the Royal Society of Medicine endorses that organisation.

Most of the organisations listed are dependent on voluntary fund-raising, occasionally supplemented by grants from central or local government. Generally, entries have been restricted to organisations which are countrywide in nature, or which are regarded as leading bodies in their field, or which welcome enquiries from anywhere in the country.

Contents

Key to symbols used in this directory

C	Charity
	Branches
	Volunteers
	Telephone advice
	Written advice
	Counselling
	Advocacy
	Information leaflets
NEWS	Newsletter
	Books/others

A

Abbeyfield Society

Abbeyfield House
53 Victoria Street
St. Albans
Hertfordshire
AL1 3UW

Admin tel: 01727 857536
Admin fax: 01727 846168

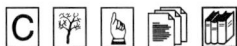

C 🌳 👆 📑 📖

Description: Provides care and companionship for older people, by providing supportive, very sheltered housing for small groups of residents living as a 'family'. Extra care is offered for larger groups of frail, older people as a 24 hour personal service provided by professional staff.

Index keyword: Elderly:
Accommodation/Housing

Able Community Care

69–75 Thorpe Road
Norwich
Norfolk
NR1 1UA

Helpline tel: **01603 764567**
Admin tel: 01603 764567
Admin fax: 01603 761655

📞 📑 NEWS

Description: Enables elderly and disabled people to continue living in their own homes, by providing a rotational live-in home-carer service. Nation-wide coverage.

Index keyword: Disability: General
Information

Abortion Law Reform Association

2–12 Pentonville Road
London
N1 9FP

Admin tel: 020 7278 5539
Admin fax: 020 7278 5239
E-mail: alra@mailbox.co.uk

🧪 📑 NEWS

Description: The Association campaigns for a woman's right to choose on abortion, both in law and in practice.

Index keyword: Abortion

Abuse in Therapy and Counselling Support Network

c/o Women's Support Project
31 Stockwell Street
Glasgow
G1 4RZ

Helpline tel: **0141 552 2221**
Admin fax: 0141 552 1876
E-mail: info@wsproject.demon.co.uk
Opening times: 10am–4.30pm

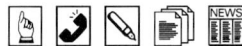

👆 📞 ✏️ 📑 NEWS

Description: Provides confidential support and information for women who have been abused within a therapeutic relationship. There is a contact list for women wishing to be put in touch with other survivors.

Index keyword: Counselling

Accept Services

724 Fulham Road
London
SW6 5SE

Helpline tel: 020 7371 7477
Admin tel: 020 7371 7455
Opening times: Mon–Wed 9am–5pm,
Thurs 12pm–6pm, Fri 9am–5pm

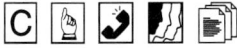

Description: Facilitators assist group
members towards understanding the
feelings and personal issues that have
played a part in problems with alcohol.

Index keyword: Alcohol Problems

Acne Support Group, The

PO Box 230
Hayes
Middlesex
UB4 0UT

Helpline tel: 020 8561 6868
Fax: 020 8845 5424
Website: www.stopspots.org
Opening times: 10am–5pm

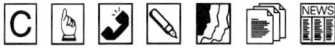

Description: Provides support to sufferers;
shows them that they are not alone.

Index keyword: Skin Problems

Acorns Childrens Hospice

Acorns Childrens Hospice Trust
103 Oak Tree Lane, Selly Oak
Birmingham
West Midlands
B29 6HZ

Helpline tel: 0121 248 4850
Admin tel: 0121 248 4800
Admin fax: 0121 248 4883

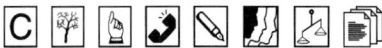

Description: Provides care and support to
life limited children and their carers.

Index keyword: Children: General
Information

Across Trust, The

Bridge House
70/72 Bridge Road
East Molesey
Surrey
KT8 9HF

Helpline tel: 020 8783 1355
Admin tel: 020 8783 1355
Admin fax: 020 8783 1622
Opening hours 8.00am–6.00pm

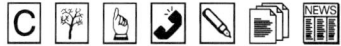

Description: Provides accompanied
holidays and pilgrimages across Europe
for persons who are terminally ill, sick or
disabled. All persons travel by
Jumbulance, a purpose-built jumbo-
ambulance, with volunteer helpers,
including qualified medical staff, on
board. Organised groups and individuals
welcome to apply.

Index keyword: Disability: Care
Scheme/Holidays

Action 19 Plus

c/o Campaigns Department
SCOPE
12 Park Crescent
London
W1N 4EQ

Admin fax: 020 7436 2601

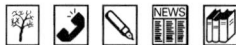

Description: Aims to empower disabled
adults, their carers, parents and other
advocates, by joint initiative, including
training, education and the dissemination

of information. Negotiates, lobbies and campaigns for good quality personal support and community care services.

Index keyword: Disability: General Information

Action Against Allergy (AAA)

PO Box 278
Twickenham
Middlesex
TW1 4QQ

Admin tel: 020 8892 2711

C 👆 ✎ 🦶 📄 NEWS 📖

Description: Provides information and guidance regarding allergic illness and advice on where specialist help can be obtained.

Index keyword: Allergies

Action Against Breast Cancer

B363 Curie Avenue
Harwell International Business Centre
Oxon
OX11 0RA

Helpline tel: **01235 820777**
Admin tel: 01235 820777
Admin fax: 01235 820506
E-mail: info@aabc.org.uk
Opening hours: 9am–5pm

C 🌳 👆 📞 📄 NEWS

Description: Raises money for new research into breast cancer, particularly to understand secondary spread. Research groups at the University College London and Middlesex Hospitals aims to identify tumour, patient and environment factors that determine long survival.

Index keyword: Cancer

Action Asthma Patient Service

Allen and Hanburys Limited
Freepost, 69 Campus Road
Listerhills Science Park
Bradford
BD7 1BR

Helpline tel: **020 8990 3011; 020 8990 2430**

📞 📄 NEWS

Description: Provides an information service for asthma sufferers

Index keyword: Asthma

Action for Dysphasic Adults (ADA)

1 Royal Street
London
SE1 7LL

Helpline tel: **020 7261 9572**
Admin tel: 020 7261 9572
Admin fax: 020 7928 9542
Opening times: 10.00am–4.00pm

C 🌳 👆 📞 📞 ✎ 🦶 🔨 📄
NEWS 📖

Description: ADA works to relieve the frustration and social isolation of people who are usually otherwise intellectually unimpaired. All forms of communication may be affected: speech, reading, writing and sometimes gesture.

Index keyword: Disability: General Information

Action for ME

PO Box 1302
Wells
Somerset
BA5 2WE

Helpline tel: **0891 122976**
Admin tel: 01749 670799
Admin fax: 01749 672561

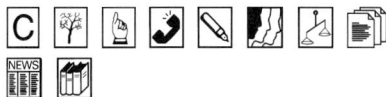

C 🌳 ☝ 📞 ✏️ 👣 📐 📑
NEWS 📖

Description: Provides advice and support to ME sufferers and their carers. Membership services include counselling lines, welfare benefits information, therapy advice, lists of sympathetic doctors, factsheets, books and a thrice-yearly journal.

Index keyword: ME (Myalgic Encephalomyelitis)

Action for Sick Children

300 Kingston Road
London
SW20 8LX

Helpline tel: **020 8542 4848**
Admin fax: 020 8542 2424

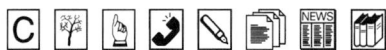

C 🌳 ☝ 📞 ✏️ 📑 NEWS 📖

Description: This is a national charity dedicated to improving the standards and quality of child healthcare in hospital, at home and in the community.

Index keyword: Childcare

Action for Sick Children (Scotland) (NAWCH)

15 Smith's Place
Edinburgh
EH6 8NT
Opening hrs 9–1 pm
Helpline tel: 0131 553 6553
Admin tel: 0131 553 6553
Admin fax: 0131 553 6553
Opening hours: 9.30am–11.30am, Mon–Fri

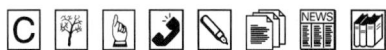

C 🌳 ☝ 📞 ✏️ 📑 NEWS 📖

Description: The principal object of Action for Sick Children is the promotion of a high standard of care for sick children at home and in hospital. It supports sick children and their families and works to ensure that health services are planned for them. It joins parents and professionals in promoting high quality health care.

Index keyword: Childcare

Action for Victims of Medical Accidents

44 High Street
1 London Road,
Croydon
Surrey
CR0 1YB

Helpline tel: **020 8686 8333**
Admin tel: 020 8686 8333
Admin fax: 020 8667 9065
Opening hours: 9.30am–5.30pm, Mon–Fri

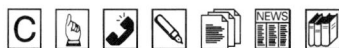

C ☝ 📞 ✏️ 📑 NEWS 📖

Description: To help people who have suffered as a result of medical treatment or the failure to give medical treatment. In addition: working for change in the attitudes of health carers towards victims and in procedures for ensuring accountability and obtaining redress.

Index keyword: Care, Support, Advice, Counselling, Bereavement, Rights, Medical, Death, Campaigning

Action on Elder Abuse

Astral House
1268 London Road
London
SW16 4ER

Helpline tel: **020 8679 7074**
Admin tel: 020 8764 7648
Admin fax: 020 8679 4074
10–4.30 pm opening hrs.

C [icons]

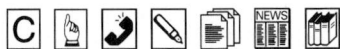

Description: Aims to prevent abuse in old age by promoting changes in policy and practice, through raising awareness, education, promoting research and the provision of information. Offers a national information service for all enquirers, a membership service, and a confidential helpline for anyone concerned about the abuse of an older person.

Index keyword: Elderly: General Information

Action on Pre-Eclampsia (APEC)

31–33 College Road
Harrow
Middlesex
HA1 1EJ

Helpline tel: 020 8427 4217
Admin tel: 020 8863 3271
Admin fax: 020 8424 0653
Website: www.apec.org.uk.
E-mail: info@apec.org.uk
Opening hours: 10.00am–1.00pm

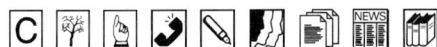

C [icons]

Description: Informs and educates parents and health professionals about pre-eclampsia; supports sufferers and their families; promotes and publicises relevant research.

Index keyword: Pregnancy and Childbirth

Action on Smoking and Health (ASH)

109 Gloucester Place
London
W1H 4EJ

Admin tel: 020 7935 3519
Admin fax: 020 7935 3463

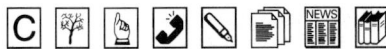

C [icons]

Description: ASH is a charity set up in 1971 by the Royal College of Physicians of London. ASH aims to work with others to eliminate the single largest preventable cause of death and disease within the UK by influencing policy and public opinion on tobacco use.

Index keyword: Smoking

Action Research

Vincent House
Horsham
West Sussex
RH12 2DP

Admin tel: 01403 210406
Admin fax: 01403 210541

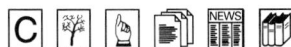

C [icons]

Description: Action Research is a charity dedicated to the prevention or treatment of disease or disability by funding vital medical research.

Index keyword: Research

AD/HD Family Support Groups UK

1a High Street
Dilton Marsh
Westbury
Wiltshire
BA13 4DL

Helpline tel: 01380 726710
Admin tel: 01373 826045
Admin fax: 01373 825158

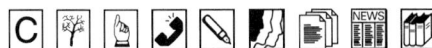

C [icons]

Description: The Attention Deficit Hyperactivity Disorder Family Support Groups UK aims to promote awareness; remove isolation; assist with issues such as medical, educational, social services, benefits; link up families. Provides free information. Organises conferences, seminars and workshops.

Index keyword: Childcare

ADA Reading Service for the Blind

6 Dalewood Rise
Laverstock
Salisbury
Wiltshire
SP1 1SF

Helpline tel: **01722 326987**
Admin tel: 01722 326987

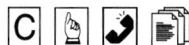

[C] [icon] [icon] [icon]

Description: Client makes initial enquiry and then provides written or printed material, together with cassettes on which the work is to be recorded (cassettes may be provided, by arrangement). The material is sent out under an 'articles for the blind' label.

Index keyword: Blindness/Visual Handicap
WORK FROM HOME OPEN ALL DAY ALL NIGHT.

Description: Aims to increase awareness of Adams-Oliver syndrome.

Index keyword: Adams-Oliver Syndrome

Addisons Disease Self Help Group

21 George Road
Guildford
GU1 4NP

Helpline tel: **01483 830673**
Admin tel: 01483 830673
Admin fax: 01483 830673

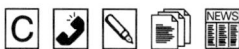

[C] [icon] [icon] [icon] [NEWS]

Description: Aims to put fellow sufferers in touch with each other.

Index keyword: Addison's Disease

Advice Service Capability Scotland (ASCS)

11 Ellersby Road
Edinburgh
EH12 6HY

Helpline tel: **0131 313 5510**
Admin tel: 0131 313 5510
Admin fax: 0131 346 1681

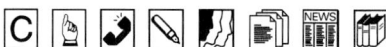

[C] [icon] [icon] [icon] [icon] [icon] [NEWS] [icon]

Description: The advice and information service provides: an enquiry service by telephone, letter, drop-in or home visit; a library, which includes books, videos, cassettes and journals; a range of information, which is produced in-house; a wide range of leaflets on cerebral palsy and related topics (eg finance, therapy, respite).

Index keyword: Cerebral Palsy

Advisory Centre for Education

1b Aberdeen Studios
22 Highbury Grove
London
N5 2DQ

Helpline tel: **020 7354 8321**
Admin tel: 020 7354 8318
Admin fax: 020 7354 9069
Opening times: 2.00am–5.00pm

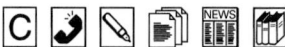

[C] [icon] [icon] [icon] [NEWS] [icon]

Description: The Advisory Centre for Education (ACE) is an independent national advice centre for parents. It runs a telephone helpline, answers letters, produces publications and offers training on all aspects of school matters, including education law. It has particular expertise on special needs, including the new code of practice.

Index keyword: Education

Advisory Committee for the Elderly and Disabled (DIEL)

50 Ludgate Hill
London
EC4M 7JJ

Helpline tel: 020 7634 8773
Admin tel: 020 7634 5301
Admin fax: 020 7634 8924
Website: www.acts.org.uk
E-mail: diel@acts.org.uk
Opening times: 9am–5pm

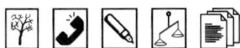

Description: DIEL is an independent advisory committee established by Act of Parliament to advise OFTEL, the telecoms regulator, on the interests and needs of consumers who happen to be either disabled or elderly, or both.

Index keyword: Disabled/Elderly

Advisory Service & Alcohol

25 the Tything
Worcester
WR1 1JL

Helpline tel: 01905 27417
Admin tel: 01905 27417
Admin fax: 01905 616517

Website: www.users.zetnet.co.uk/hwasa/
E-mail: wasa@btclick.com
Opening times: 9am–5pm, Mon–Fri

Description: Offers one-to-one counselling to drinkers and anyone affected.

Aftermath

PO Box 414
Sheffield
S1 3UP

Helpline tel: 0114 2758520

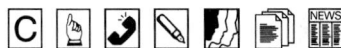

Description: Aftermath offers support and counselling to the families of serious offenders.

Index keyword: Counselling

Age Concern Cymru

1 Cathedral Road
Cardiff
CF11 9SD

Admin tel: 029 2037 1566
Fax no: 029 2039 9562
Website: www.accymru.org.uk
E-mail: enquiries@accymru.org.uk

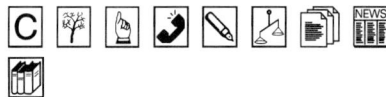

Description: Age Concern has been working for over 50 years to ensure that older people receive the support, the encouragement and, where necessary, the care they need to make life as enjoyable and rewarding as it can be.

Index keyword: Elderly: General Information

Age Concern England

Astral House
1268 London Road
London
SW16 4ER

Helpline **0800 009966**
Admin tel: 020 8765 7200
Admin fax: 020 8765 7211
Website: www.ace.org.uk
E-mail: ace@ace.org.uk
Opening hours: 7.00am–7.30pm

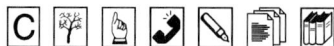

Description: Age Concern England, the National Council on Ageing, is the centre of a network of 1,100 local organisations which offer a wide range of community-based services, including day centres, home visiting and transport. Nationally, Age Concern supports this work through provision of information and advice, policy analysis, publications, grants, training and campaigning.

Index keyword: Elderly: General Information

Age Concern Scotland

113 Rose Street
Edinburgh
EH2 3DT

Admin tel: 0131 220 3345
Admin fax: 0131 220 2779
E-mail: enquiries@acsinfo3.freeserve.co.uk

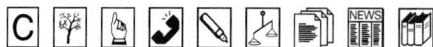

Description: Works throughout Scotland to ensure that all older people have their rights addressed, their voices heard and have choice and control over all aspects of their lives.

Index keyword: Elderly: General Information

Aids Care Education and Training (ACET)

PO Box 3693
London
SW15 2BQ

Helpline tel: **020 7511 0110**
Admin tel: 020 8780 0400
Admin fax: 020 8780 0450
Website: www.acetuk.org
E-mail: acet@acetuk.org

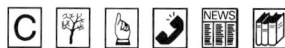

Description: In communities around the world, ACET provides unconditional care for those with HIV/AIDS, and practical education and training about HIV and its prevention. Worldwide, ACET supports and co-operates with others who are responding to AIDS in their community. ACET works with national and international agencies to promote policies to reduce the spread of HIV.

Index keyword: AIDS and HIV

Air Transport Users Council

CAA House
45–59 Kingsway
London
WC2B 6TE

Admin tel: 020 7240 6061
Admin fax: 020 7240 7071
Website: www.auc.org.uk

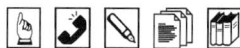

Description: This is an independent body, with members throughout the UK, which looks after the interests of all airline passengers, whether they are travelling on business or for pleasure.

Index keyword: General Information

Al-Anon Family Groups UK and Eire

61 Great Dover Street
London
SE1 4YF

Helpline tel: **020 7403 0888**
Admin fax: 020 7378 9910
Website: www.hexnet.co.uk/alanon
E-mail: alanonuk@aol.com
Opening times: 24 hours 7 days week

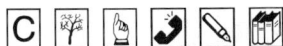

[C] [tree] [hand] [phone] [pencil] [book]

Description: Al-Anon is a worldwide fellowship for families and friends of problem drinkers. There are over 1000 self-help groups in the UK and Eire. Alateen is part of Al-Anon for teenagers with an alcoholic relative. Please ring for details of local meetings.

Index keyword: Alcohol Problems

Al-Anon Information Centre

Room 338
Baltic Chambers
50 Wellington Street
Glasgow
G2 6HJ

Helpline tel: **0141 221 7356**
Admin tel: 0141 221 7356
Opening times: 10am–4pm Mon–Fri (answerphone other times)

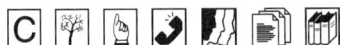

[C] [tree] [hand] [phone] [foot] [pages] [book]

Description: Al-Anon's sole purpose is to help families of problem drinkers.

Index keyword: Alcohol Problems

Albany Trust

Art of Health and Yoga
280 Balham High Road
London
SW17 7AL

Helpline tel: **020 8767 1827**
Admin tel: 020 8767 1827

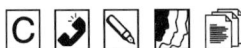

[C] [phone] [pencil] [foot] [pages]

Description: Counsellors are trained and experienced in working with relationship and marital difficulties, communication problems and sex therapy. Counselling around sexual identity and experiences of sexual abuse; gender orientation; HIV and AIDS-related psychological issues. They offer one-to-one counselling; couples work; family therapy; and group work.

Index keyword: Sexual Problems

Alcohol Concern

Waterbridge House
32–36 Loman Street
London
SE1 0EE

Helpline tel: **020 7928 7377**
Admin tel: 020 7928 7377
Admin fax: 020 7928 4644

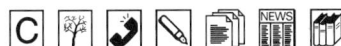

[C] [tree] [phone] [pencil] [pages] [NEWS] [book]

Description: Aims to reduce the costs of alcohol misuse and to develop the range and quality of services available to problem drinkers and their families. Activities include service development, policy, library, publications and a workplace advisory service.

Index keyword: Alcohol Problems

Alcohol Counselling and Prevention Services

34 Electric Lane
London
SW9 8JT

Admin tel: 020 7737 3579
Admin fax: 020 7737 2719
Website: www.vois.org.uk/acaps
E-mail: acaps.uk@virgin.net

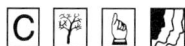

Description: The service provides education about sensible drinking, training (London-wide) and counselling for individuals, couples and groups, with a choice of counsellors.

Index keyword: Alcohol Problems

Alcohol Recovery Project

68 Newington Causeway
Elephant & Castle
London
SE1 6DF

Admin tel: 020 7403 3369
Admin fax: 020 7357 6712
Website: www.arp-charity.demon.co.uk/arp.htm
E-mail: arp-charity.demon.co.uk

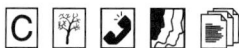

Description: Offers counselling, advice, social work and housing services to people with a history of alcohol dependency.

Index keyword: Alcohol Problems

Alcoholics Anonymous (London Region Telephone Service)

2nd Floor
Jacob House

3–5 Cynthia Street
London
N1 9JE

Helpline tel: **020 7833 0022**
Opening times: 10am–10pm

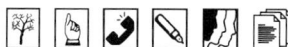

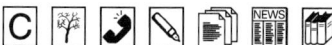

Description: Aims to put everyone who wishes to stop drinking in touch with their local Alcoholics Anonymous group.

Index keyword: Alcohol Problems

Alcoholics Anonymous

PO Box 1, Stonebow House
Stonebow
York
North Yorkshire
YO1 7NJ

Helpline tel: **020 7833 0022**
Admin tel: 01904 644026
Admin fax: 01904 629091
Website: www.alcoholics-anonymous.org.uk
Opening times: 10am–10pm

Description: Alcoholics Anonymous is a fellowship of men and women who share their experience, strength and hope with one another, so that they may solve their common problem and help others to recover from alcoholism. The only requirement for membership is a desire to stop drinking.

Index keyword: Alcohol Problems

Aled Richards Trust

8–10 West Street
Old Market
Bristol
BS2 0BH

Admin tel: 0117 955 1000

Admin fax: 0117 954 1200
E-mail: info@aled-richards-trust.org.uk

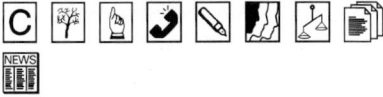

[icons]

Description: The trust offers care and support to all people affected by HIV and AIDS in the West of England. Services include buddying, counselling, complementary therapies, advice and information, health promotion, drop in centre, support groups, financial help, Peer led treatment.

Index keyword: AIDS and HIV

Aleph One Limited

The Old Courthouse
Bottisham
Cambridge
CB5 9BA

Admin tel: 01223 811679
Admin fax: 01223 812713
Website: www.aleph1.co.uk
E-mail: info@aleph1.co.uk

[icons]

Description: Supplies aids for stress management, including audio-cassettes on relaxation and particular behavioural problems; books useful to sufferers and to those who help them; and biofeedback instruments to enable sufferers, with or without the aid of a therapist, to understand and control their stress, muscle tension, etc.

Index keyword: Stress

Alexander Technique International

142 Thorpedale Road
London
N4 3BS

Admin fax: 020 7281 9400

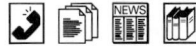

[icons]

Description: Alexander lessons can benefit people who suffer from chronic pain or injury (back injury, for instance), as well as musicians, performers etc, who want to be able to perform with greater ease. ATI is a professional society; all teachers listed are qualified Alexander teachers.

Index keyword: Holistic

Alliance for Cannabis Therapeutics (ACT)

PO Box CR14
Leeds
L57 4XF

Admin fax: 0113 237 1000

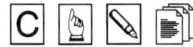

[icons]

Description: Campaigns to have cannabis made available on prescription for seriously ill patients whom it would help. Please send four first class stamps for information.

Index keyword: Complementary Medicine

Alzheimer Scotland (Action on Dementia)

22 Drumsheugh Gardens
Edinburgh
EH3 7RN

Helpline tel: 0808 808 3000 24 hours
Admin tel: 0131 243 1453
Admin fax: 0131 243 1450
Website: www.alzscot.org
E-mail: alzheimer@alzscot.org
Opening times: 24 hours (7 days)

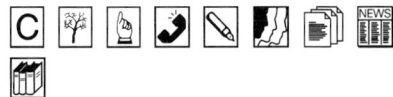

[icons]

Description: Alzheimer Scotland helps people with dementia, their carers and families. Our members, who are individual carers, social workers, care workers, doctors, groups and organisations interested in dementia, share our aims: to be the national voice of people with dementia and their carers; to improve public policies; to provide and secure high quality services.

Index keyword: Alzheimers Disease

Alzheimers Disease Society

Gordon House
10 Greencoat Place
London
SW1P 1PH

Helpline tel: 0845 3000 336
Admin tel: 020 7306 0606
Admin fax: 020 7306 0808
Website: www.alzheimers.org.uk
E-mail: info@alzheimers.org.uk

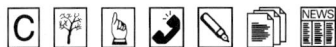

Description: Supports families and professionals caring for someone with Alzheimer's disease or other forms of dementia.

Index keyword: Alzheimers Disease

Alzheimers Disease Society (Northern Ireland)

86 Aglantine Avenue
Belfast
BT9 6EU

Helpline tel: 028 9066 4100
Admin tel: 028 9066 4100
Admin fax: 028 9066 4440
Opening times: 9am–5pm

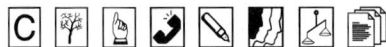

Description: The Alzheimer's Disease Society is the leading care and research charity for people with dementia. It provides information and education, support for carers, and quality day and home care. It funds medical and scientific research, campaigns for improved health and social services, and greater public understanding of dementia.

Index keyword: Alzheimers Disease

Amnesty International UK

99–119 Rosebery Avenue
London
EC1R 4RE

Admin tel: 020 7814 6200
Admin fax: 020 7833 1510
Website: www.amnesty.org.uk
E-mail: info@amnesty.org.uk

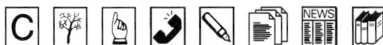

Description: Campaigns on behalf of prisoners who are tortured or given inadequate medical treatment. Campaigns for the release of prisoners of conscience. Involved in education, advice and campaigns to stop torture, the death penalty and human rights abuses.

Index keyword: General Information

Anaphylaxis Campaign

PO Box 149
Fleet
Hampshire
GU13 0FA

Admin tel: 01252 542029
Admin fax: 01252 377140
Website: www.anaphylaxis.org.uk

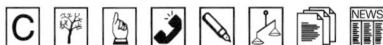

Description: Aims to raise awareness of potentially fatal food allergies and to provide information and guidance to sufferers.

Index keyword: Allergies

Androgen Insensitivity Support Group

PO Box 269
Banbury
Oxfordshire
OX15 8YT

Only for Patient: 01295 670140

The Angel Drug Services

Arena House
66–68 Pentonville Road
Islington
London
N19 HS

Helpline tel: **24 hours 0800 169 2679;**
Client line: 020 7833 4181
Admin tel: 020 7833 9899
Admin fax: 020 7833 1419
Opening hours: 10.00am–5.30pm

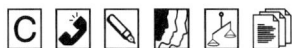

[C] [☎] [✎] [👣] [⚖] [📄]

Description: The Angel Drug Services is an independent voluntary sector organisation based in Islington, working with individuals and community groups affected by legal and illegal drug use.

The services exists to reduce the harmful effects of drug use for users, their families and friends, as well as for the community as a whole.

Index keyword: Drug Addiction/Side Effects

Angelman Syndrome Support Group

15 Place Crescent
Waterlooville
Hampshire
PO7 5UR

Helpline tel: **023 9238 5566**
Admin tel: 023 9226 4224
Admin fax: 023 9224 1977

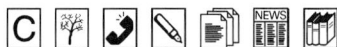

[C] [🌳] [☎] [✎] [📄] [NEWS] [📰]

Description: Provides support and information to families and carers of Angelman Syndrome children and adults. Encourages local area family contact and produces newsletters. There are also regional meetings and a bi-annual conference. A booklet and video are available.

Index keyword: Angelman Syndrome

Ante-Natal Results and Choices (ARC)

73 Charlotte Street
London
W1T 4PN

Helpline tel: **020 7631 0285**
Admin tel: 020 7631 0280
Admin fax: 020 7631 0280

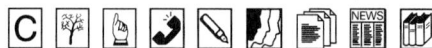

[C] [🌳] [👆] [☎] [✎] [👣] [📄] [NEWS] [📰]

Description: SAFTA helps parents who discover that their unborn baby may have an abnormality.

Index keyword: Pregnancy and Childbirth

Anthony Nolan Bone Marrow Trust, The

The Royal Free Hospital
Pond Street
Hampstead
London
NW3 2QG

Helpline tel: **020 7284 1234**
Admin fax: 020 7284 8226

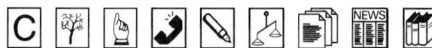

[C] [🌳] [👆] [☎] [✎] [⚖] [📄] [NEWS] [📰]

Description: Provides unrelated bone marrow donors for patients suffering from leukaemia and other allied bone marrow disorders, regardless of race, colour or creed. The trust also undertakes research into improving the outcome of bone marrow transplantation.

Index keyword: Bone Marrow

A

Anxiety and Phobia Network

4 Randu Road
Cricklewood
London
NW2 3HA

Description: Provides information on therapies (conventional and alternative) for anxiety and phobias.

Index keyword: Phobias

Anything Left-Handed Limited

18 Avenue Road
Belmont
Surrey
SM2 6JD

Helpline tel: 020 8770 3722
Admin fax: 020 8715 1220

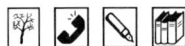

Description: Established for over 25 years, this is the leading supplier of left-handed products, eg scissors, tin-openers, corkscrews and pens (over 200 products available). Left-Handers Club formed in 1990. Keeps members in touch with developments, promotes research and offers discount on left-handed items.

Index keyword: Lefthanded

Appropriate Health Resources and Technologies Action Group (AHRTAG)

40 Adler Street
London
E1 1EE

Admin tel: 020 7539 1570
Admin fax: 020 7539 1580

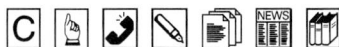

Description: AHRTAG is committed to strengthening primary health care and community based rehabilitation in the south by maximising the use and impact of information, providing training and resources, and actively supporting the capacity-building of partner organisations.

Index keyword: General Health

Arbours Association Limited

6 Church Lane
London
N8 7BU

Helpline tel: 020 8340 7646
Admin tel: 020 8340 7646
Admin fax: 020 8341 5822

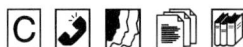

Description: Aims to provide therapeutic living environments as an alternative to psychiatric hospitals. Runs three long-stay households, a short-stay crisis centre, and a psychotherapy clinic, including low cost therapy where appropriate. All facilities are located in the London area.

Index keyword: Mental Health/Illness

ARP Choices (black advisory services for alcohol-related concerns)

140 Stockwell Road
London
SW9 9TQ

Admin tel: 020 7737 3363; 020 7737 0393
Admin fax: 020 7737 5755

C ▢ ▢ ☎ ✎ ▢ ▢ ▢

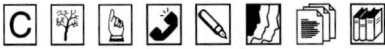

Description: Aims to target ARP Choices services to the black community in Lambeth, Southwark, Lewisham and London-wide. Provides advice/counselling and support to people with alcohol-related concerns in one-to-one and group settings; outreach work in surgeries or other settings; free complementary therapies.

Index keyword: Alcohol Problems

Arthritic Association

1st Floor Suite
2 Hyde Gardens
Eastbourne
East Sussex
BN21 4PN

Helpline tel: **020 7491 0233**
Admin tel: 020 7491 0233
Admin fax: 01323 639793

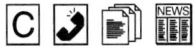

C ☎ ▢ ▢

Description: Helps people who are suffering or who have suffered from arthritis, or any allied illness, to regain freedom from pain and enjoy a more healthy life, abundant with energy. They provide items, services or facilities to alleviate suffering and assist recovery.

Index keyword: Arthritis/Rheumatic Disorders

Arthritis Care

18 Stephenson Way
London
NW1 2HD

Helpline tel: **0800 289170**
Admin tel: 020 7916 1500
Admin fax: 020 7916 1505

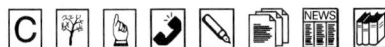

C ▢ ▢ ☎ ✎ ▢ ▢ ▢

Description: For nearly 50 years, Arthritis Care has been working with people with arthritis to promote their health, well-being and independence through services, support, self-help, information and influence. It has 650 branches and groups throughout England, Scotland, Wales and Northern Ireland.

Index keyword: Arthritis/Rheumatic Disorders

ASG

Canterbury House
1–3 Greengate
Salford
Manchester
M3 7NN

Helpline tel: **0800 616101 (freephone)**
Admin tel: 0161 839 8442
Admin fax: 0161 834 5850

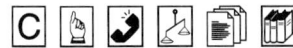

C ▢ ☎ ▢ ▢ ▢

Description: Provides an independent and confidential advocacy service to children and young people living away from home.

Index keyword: Childcare

Ashwellthorpe Hall Association

Ashwellthorpe Hall Hotel
The Street
Ashwellthorpe, Norwich
Norfolk
NR16 1EX

Helpline tel: **01508 489324**
Admin tel: 01508 489324
Admin fax: 01508 488409
Opening times: Any time

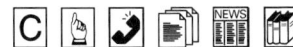

C ▢ ☎ ▢ ▢ ▢

Description: The association is a charity specialising in affordable holidays for people with disabilities, their family and friends. Set in 15 acres of grounds, the hotel is entirely wheelchair-friendly. Aids include fitted hoists, electric beds, closomat toilets etc. There is an adapted mini-bus with tail-lift for trips out. Links are maintained with care agencies.

Index keyword: Disability: Care Scheme/Holidays

Asian Family Counselling Service

74 The Avenue
West Ealing
London
W13 8LB

Admin tel: 020 8997 5749
Admin fax: 020 8998 1880

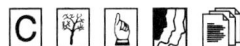

[C] [tree] [hand] [face] [docs]

Description: The service provides marital and family counselling for the Asian community.

Index keyword: Ethnic Minorities

Aspire

RNOHT
Brockley Hill
Stanmore
Middlesex
HA7 4LP

Admin tel: 020 8954 0701
Admin fax: 020 8420 6352

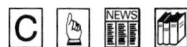

[C] [hand] [NEWS] [book]

Description: Aspire exists to raise funds and support projects that will enable people who have sustained a spinal cord injury, and disabled people generally, to lead fulfilled and independent lives.

Index keyword: Spinal Injuries

Association for Brain Damaged Children and Young Adults, The

Clifton House
3 St Paul's Road, Foleshill
Foleshill
Coventry
CV6 5DE

Helpline tel: **024 7666 5450**
Admin tel: 024 7666 5450
Admin fax: 024 7666 5450 (phone beforehand)
Opening times: 9.30am–1.30pm

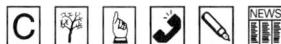

[C] [tree] [hand] [phone] [pencil] [NEWS]

Description: ABDC provides a residential home for adults and a respite home for children with learning difficulties. Strives to assist each young person to reach his or her own potential in a supportive and caring environment in partnership with their families and schools.

Index keyword: Brain Injuries

Association for Children with Heart Disorders, The

Killieard House
Killiecrankie
Pitlochry
Perthshire
PH16 5LN

Helpline tel: **01796 473204**
Admin tel: 01796 473204
Admin fax: 01796 473204

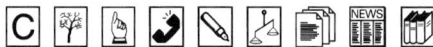

[C] [tree] [hand] [phone] [pencil] [flask] [docs] [NEWS] [book]

Description: Gives support and understanding in everyday care and welfare to parents and families of children with heart disorders. Raises money for research into congenital heart disorders and helps children's heart units improve facilities and maintain improvements in hospitals as new techniques develop. Provides weekend breaks for young adults and families.

Index keyword: Heart Problems

Association for Children with Life-Threatening or Terminating Conditions and their families (ACT)

65 St Michael's Hill
Bristol
BS2 8DZ

Admin tel: 0117 922 1556
Admin fax: 0117 930 4707

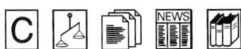

C ⚗ 🗐 NEWS 📊

Description: ACT aims to inform families about available services, in both the statutory and voluntary sectors, through its national database and literature resource. It supports people who are planning and providing children's hospices and other services in the community, and organises national conferences and seminars.

Index keyword: Childcare

Association for Cushings Treatment and Help

54 Powney Road
Maidenhead
Berkshire
SL6 6EQ

Helpline tel: **01628 670389**
Admin tel: 01628 670389
Admin fax: 01628 415603
E-mail: cushingsacth@btinternet.com

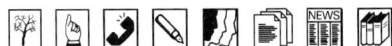

🌳 👆 ☎ ✎ 🦵 🗐 NEWS 📊

Description: The Association aims to help and support new and longer-standing sufferers from Cushing's Syndrome, as a resource for easing their experience

during diagnosis, treatment and follow-up, and helping them to recover the best possible quality of life.

Index keyword: Cushing Syndrome

Association for Glycogen Storage Disease, The (UK)

9 Lindop Road
Hale
Altrincham
Cheshire
WA15 9DZ

Helpline tel: **0161 980 7303**
Admin tel: 0161 980 7303
Admin fax: 0161 226 3813

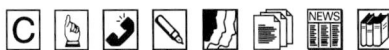

C 👆 ☎ ✎ 🦵 🗐 NEWS 📊

Description: The AGSD(UK) acts primarily as a family contact and support group for all persons affected by GSD. It also aims to encourage the provision of specialist centres for the diagnosis, monitoring and treatment of GSD persons, both children and adults, and to act as a focus for scientific, educational and charitable activities concerning GSD.

Index keyword: General Information

Association of Humanistic Psychology

BCM AHPP
London
WC1N 3XX

Admin tel: 0845 7660326
Admin fax: 01348 840845

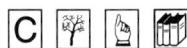

C 🌳 👆 📖

Description: AHP was formed in 1969 to promote knowledge about and the application of humanistic psychology. It runs conferences and has a practitioners' sub-group which provides accreditation for psychotherapists.

Index keyword: Psychotherapy

Association for Improvements in the Maternity Services (AIMS)

40 Kingswood Avenue
London
NW6 6LS

Helpline tel: **020 8960 5585; 01772 615840**
Admin tel: 020 8960 5585
Admin fax: 01753 654142

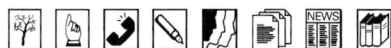

Description: AIMS was founded in 1960 and has individual members in England, Ireland, Scotland and Wales, the majority of whom are parents and midwives. AIMS offers an information service to parents. It also provides support and advice about parents' rights, complaint procedures and choices within maternity care. Acts as a campaigning pressure group for improvements in the maternity services. Supports parents in making informed choice in childbirth.

Index keyword: Pregnancy and Childbirth

Association for Residential Care

ARC House
Marsden Street
Chesterfield
Derbyshire
S40 1JY

Helpline tel: **01246 555043**
Admin tel: 01246 555043
Admin fax: 01246 555045

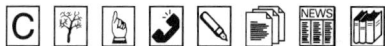

Description: Promotes the quality of life, maintenance of standards and diversity of residential and day service provision for people with a learning disability.

Index keyword: Mental Health/Illness

Association for Spina Bifida And Hydrocephalus (ASBAH)

ASBAH House
42 Park Road
Peterborough
PE1 2UQ

Admin tel: 01733 555988
Admin fax: 01733 555985

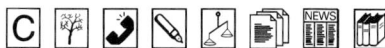

Description: Provides services for people with spina bifida and/or hydrocephalus and their carers and parents. Specialist fieldworkers cover most of England, Wales and Northern Ireland.

Index keyword: Spina Bifida

Association of Charity Officers, The

Beechwood House
Wyllyotts Close
Potters Bar
Hertfordshire
EN6 2HN

Helpline tel: **01707 651777**
Admin tel: 01707 651777
Admin fax: 01707 660477

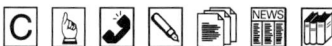

Description: Campaigns on behalf of charities in the field of benevolence and personal social welfare. ACO is consulted by government, enquiry and review bodies; gives members information and advice on key issues; keeps abreast of legislation; promotes the efficiency and effectiveness of charities; focuses on issues of concern to members

Index keyword: General Information

Association of Community Health Councils for England and Wales (ACHCEW)

30 Drayton Park
London
N5 1PB

Admin tel: 020 7609 8405
Admin fax: 020 7700 1152

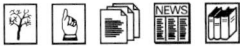

Description: Provides a forum for member CHCs, with information and advice; and represents the user of health services at a national level.

Index keyword: Patients Rights

Association of Crossroads Care Attendant Schemes Limited, The

10 Regent Place
Rugby
Warwickshire
CV21 2PN

Helpline tel: 01788 573653
Admin tel: 01788 573653
Admin fax: 01788 565498

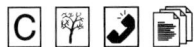

Description: Crossroads promotes, offers, supports and delivers high quality services for carers and people with care needs.

Index keyword: Carers

Association of Disabled Professionals

BCM ADP
London
WC1N 3XX

Helpline tel: 01924 283253
Admin tel: 01924 270335
Admin fax: 01924 283253

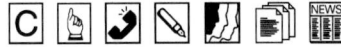

Description: Aims to improve education, rehabilitation, training and employment opportunities available to disabled people. Encourages disabled people to develop their physical and mental capacities fully, to find and retain employment commensurate with their abilities and qualifications, and to participate fully in the everyday life of society.

Index keyword: Disability: Employment

Association of Natural Medicine

27 Braintree Road
Witham
Essex
CM8 2DD

Admin tel: 01376 502762; 01376 570067
Admin fax: 01376 502762

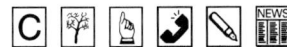

Description: Promotes the benefits of natural therapies. Runs part-time courses in homoeopathy, diet and nutrition, acupuncture, reflexology, aromatherapy, massage and counselling skills. Their clinic offers a wide range of treatments.

Index keyword: Complementary Medicine

Association of Parents of Vaccine Damaged Children

78 Campden Road
Shipston on Stour
Warwickshire
CV36 4DH

Helpline tel: 01608 661595
Admin fax: 01608 663432

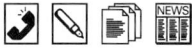

Description: The association campaigns for state compensation for vaccine damage.

Index keyword: Children: General Information

Association of Radical Midwives

62 Greetby Hill
Ormskirk
Lancashire
L39 2DT

Helpline tel: 01695 572776
Admin tel: 01695 572776
Admin fax: 01695 572776

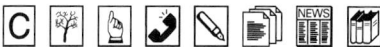

Description: Provides support and information for those having difficulty in getting or giving sympathetic, individualised NHS maternity care. Produces leaflets, *What is a midwife?* and *Choices in childbirth*. Membership is open to midwives and non-midwives. National and local meetings. Library (free loan to members). Local contacts around UK. Please send sae.

Index keyword: Pregnancy and Childbirth

Association of Therapeutic Healers

Membership Secretary
42 Braydon Road
London
N16 6QB

Description: An association for professional healers who combine healing with other therapies. Aims to promote health, well-being and self-wisdom and forum for discussion; professional referral network and register of practitioners.

Index keyword: Holistic

Association to aid the Sexual and Personal Relationships of People with a Disability, The (SPOD)

286 Camden Road
London
N7 0BJ

Helpline tel: 020 7607 8851
Admin tel: 020 7607 8851

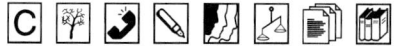

Description: Provides a direct service to people with a disability and/or their partners who are experiencing sexual or relationship problems. Also offers training and consciousness-raising work for professional carers.

Index keyword: Disability: General Information

Ataxia

10 Winchester House
Kennington Park
Cranmer Road
London
SW9 6EJ

Helpline tel: 020 7582 1444
Admin fax: 020 7582 9444

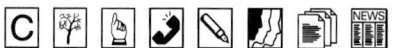

Description: Raises money for research into ataxia and provides information, advice and support to sufferers, their families and carers. Offers a limited care services fund.

Index keyword: General Information

Attia Research Trust into ALD

36 Baker Street
London
W1M 1DG

Helpline tel: 020 7580 5089
Admin fax: 020 7224 0681

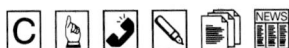

Description: The trust aims to further medical research into ALD (adrenoleukodystrophy); to help and support families with affected children; to provide home respite care; to raise public awareness of the condition.

Index keyword: General Information

AVERT (AIDS Education and Research Trust, The)

11 Denne Parade
Horsham
West Sussex
RH12 1JD

Admin tel: 01403 210202
Admin fax: 01403 211001

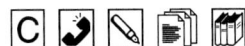

Description: Works to prevent people becoming infected with HIV, to improve the quality of life for people already infected and to work with others towards a cure. AVERT has won international recognition for its work in AIDS research and education.

Index keyword: AIDS and HIV

Avon Tyrrell Residential Centre

Bransgore
Hampshire
BH23 8EE

Admin tel: 01425 672347
Admin fax: 01425 673883

Description: This is a residential activity centre for groups of up to 120. Dormitory accommodation, fully catered, situated in the new forest, Hampshire. Facilities for disabled people.

Index keyword: Disability: Care Scheme/Holidays

Ayurvedic Company of Great Britain

81 Wimpole Street
London
W1M 7DB

Admin tel: 020 7370 2255
Admin fax: 020 7224 6080

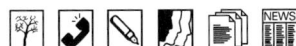

Description: Promotes the ayurvedic system of medicine by providing traditional ayurvedic treatments for several ailments, such as arthritis, gastro-intestinal and liver disorders, lumbago, sciatica, skin diseases, stress etc. The company is actively involved in co-ordinating research work and development with respect to natural products and has a comprehensive herbal database.

Index keyword: Complementary Medicine

Baby Life Support Systems (BLISS)

2nd Floor, Camalsord House
87–89 Albert Embankment
London
SE1 7TP

Helpline tel: 0500 618140
Admin tel: 020 7820 9471
Admin fax: 020 7820 9567
Website: www.bliss.org.uk
E-mail: information@bliss.org.uk

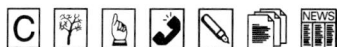

C ✡ ✍ ☎ ✎ 🖹 📰

Description: BLISS was founded to give every baby born in the UK an equal chance. To achieve this, BLISS donates life-saving equipment to neonatal units; sponsors specialist nurse training; and offers support and information to parents with babies needing specialist care at birth.

Index keyword: Childcare

The Back-Up Trust

The Business Village
Broomhill Road
London
SW18 4JQ

Helpline tel: 020 8875 1805
Admin fax: 020 8870 3619
E-mail: back-up@dialpipex.com

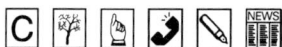

C ✡ ✍ ☎ ✎ 📰

Description: Back-up is a national charity whose aim is to encourage individuals with spinal cord injury to become reintegrated into the community and regain motivation, inspiration and independence through sporting activities.

Index keyword: Spinal Injuries

Banstead Mobility Centre

Damson Way
Orchard Hill
Fountain Drive, Carshalton
Surrey
SM5 4NR

Admin tel: 020 8770 1151
Admin fax: 020 8770 1211
Website: www.qefed.org
E-mail: mobility@banstead53.freeserve.co.uk

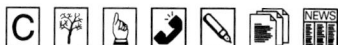

C ✡ ✍ ☎ ✎ 🖹 📰

Description: The centre provides information, assessment and training to enable disabled and elderly people achieve an optimum level of outdoor independent mobility. It publishes a list of driving instructors experienced in disability tuition.

Index keyword: Disability: General Information

Barnardo's

Tanners Lane
Barkingside
Ilford
Essex
IG6 IQG

Admin tel: 020 8550 8822
Admin fax: 020 8551 6870
Website: www.barnardos.org.uk

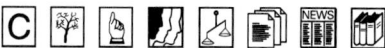

C ✡ ✍ 👣 △ 🖹 📰 📖

Description: Barnardo's works with some 47000 children, young people and families. Its 300 services provide accommodation and support for young people who are leaving care; youth training; day care in deprived areas; special education for children with disabilities; and adoption and fostering. Works with children affected by poverty, HIV/AIDS, homelessness and abuse.

Index keyword: Childcare

Beama Foundation for Disabled People

c/o RADAR
12 City Forum
250 City Road
London
ECIV 8AF

Admin tel: 020 7250 3222
Admin fax: 020 7250 0212
Website: www.radar.org.uk
E-mail: radar@radar.org.uk

Description: Aims to assist disabled persons, whether individually or collectively, through the provision of specialised equipment or apparatus (preferably electrically or electronically operated).

Index keyword: Disability: Equipment

Beaumont Society, The

27 Old Gloucester Street
London
WCIN 3XX

Helpline tel: **01582 412220**
Website: www.beaumontsociety.org.uk

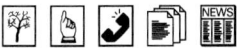

Description: A self-help organisation for people who cross-dress and their families.

Index keyword: General Information

Beckwith Wiedemann Support Group

The Drum and Monkey
Hazelbury Bryan
Dorset
DM0 2EE

Helpline tel: **0589 211000**
Admin fax: 01202 205325
E-mail: rbaker5165@aol.com

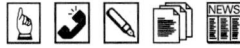

Description: Helps families of BWS-affected children. Offers advice and information.

Index keyword: Beckwith Wiedemann Syndrome

Beethoven Fund for Deaf Children, The

PO Box 16975
London
NW8 6ZL

Admin tel: 020 7722 7981
Admin fax: 020 7586 8107

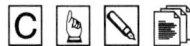

Description: Provides specially designed musical instruments to schools for deaf children; video for teachers; occasional workshops.

Index keyword: Hearing Problems/Deafness

Benefit Enquiry Line for People with Disabilities

Room 901
Victoria House
Ormskirk Road, Preston
Lancashire
PR1 2QP

Helpline tel: **0800 882200**
Admin tel: 01772 238994
Admin fax: 01772 238953
Opening times: Mon-Fri, 8.30am-6.30pm, Sat, 9am-1pm

Description: BEL provides general advice on all social security benefits and how to claim (but no access to individual records). For help in completing some benefit claim forms, phone free: 0800 441144. Textphone users: 0800 243355.

Index keyword: Disability: General Information

Bengali Workers Association

Surma Community Centre
1 Robert Street
London
NW1 3JU

Helpline tel: **020 7388 7313**
Admin tel: 020 7388 7313
Admin fax: 020 7387 8731

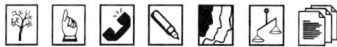

Description: As well as advice sessions, the association provides a nursery, English language classes, sewing classes, music and drama classes, Bengali classes, youth club for girls and boys, careers service, an elderly welfare project lunch club and a women's group.

Index keyword: Ethnic Minorities

Berkshire Multiple Sclerosis Therapy Centre

Bradbury House
August End
Brock Gardens
Reading
Berkshire
RG30 2JP

Helpline tel: **0118 9016000**
Admin fax: 0118 9016001

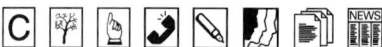

Description: Provides information, advice, support and a range of treatments aimed at managing and limiting the progression of the disease. Aims to give everyone living with MS the opportunity to access the correct information to lead a normal life.

Index keyword: Multiple Sclerosis

Birmingham Tapes for the Handicapped Association

20 Middleton Hall Road
Kings Norton
Birmingham
B30 1BY

Helpline tel: **0121 628 3656**
Admin tel: 0121 628 3656
E-mail: btha@gofornet.co.uk
Opening times: 9am–5pm

Description: The association sends out magazine tapes to disabled and elderly people, nationwide, and has a tape library which is free to members.

Index keyword: Disability: General Information

Birth Centre Limited, The

37 Coverton Road
London
SW17 0QW

Admin tel: 020 8767 8294
Admin fax: 020 8682 2275
Website: www.birthcentre.com
E-mail: midwifecf@aol.com

Description: The Birth Centre is a comfortable, private, home-like centre, where women can give birth in water, in alternative positions, or however they choose. The Birth Centre is next door to St George's Hospital in Tooting and so women can be quickly transferred there if there are any problems.

Index keyword: Pregnancy and Childbirth

Birth Defects Foundation

Martindale
Cannock
Staffs
WS11 2XN

Admin tel: 01543 4262777
Admin fax: 01543 468999
Website: www.birthdefects.co.uk
E-mail: help@birthdefects.co.uk
Opening times: 9.30am–6.00pm, Mon–Sat

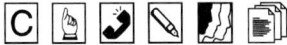

Description: Works to improve child health by the prevention and treatment of birth defects. Gives support and information to affected families.

Index keyword: Pregnancy and Childbirth

Blue Cross

Shilton Road
Burford
Oxfordshire
OX18 4PF

Admin tel: 01993 822651
Admin fax: 01993 823083
Website: www.bluecross.org.uk
E-mail: info@bluecross.org.uk

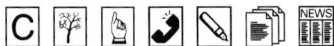

Description: Blue Cross exists to foster the bond of friendship between animals and people.

Index keyword: General Information

BNA

The Colonnades
Beaconsfield Close
Hatfield
Herts
AL10 8YD

Helpline tel: **0800 657575**
Admin tel: 01707 263544
Admin fax: 01707 272250
Website: www.bna.co.uk
E-mail: info@bna.co.uk

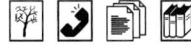

Description: BNA provides care in the community all across Britain in Hospitals, Nursing Homes, factories and offices. It also offers flexible and affordable care to people in their own homes.

Index keyword: Nursing Homes

Boarding School Survivors

128a Northview Road
London
N8 7LP

Admin tel: 020 8341 4885

Description: Provides therapeutic support, via intensive courses, for people who have been 'damaged' by boarding school education; also seeks to raise public awareness.

Index keyword: Counselling

Bobath Centre for Children with Cerebral Palsy, The

250 East End Road
East Finchley
London
N2 8AU

Admin tel: 020 8444 3355

Admin fax: 020 8444 3399
Website: www.bobathlondon.co.uk
E-mail: info@bobathlondon.co.uk

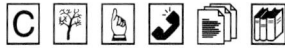

C 🌳 👆 📞 📑 📚

Description: Provides advice and treatment for children suffering from cerebral palsy; training for doctors and therapists.

Index keyword: Cerebral Palsy

Body Positive

51b Philbeach Gardens
London
SW5 9EB

Helpline tel: 020 7373 9124
Admin fax: 020 7373 5237

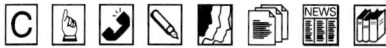

C 👆 📞 ✏️ 🦶 📑 NEWS 📚

Description: Body Positive is a self-help group providing information and support to all people living with or affected by HIV/AIDS. Facilities available include information room, helpline, hospital visiting, drop-in centre, complementary therapies, health/legal advice, monthly newsletter and support groups.

Index keyword: AIDS and HIV

Bourne Trust, The

Lincoln House
1–3 Brixton Road
London
SW9 6DE

Helpline tel: 020 7582 6699
Admin tel: 020 7582 1313
Admin fax: 020 7735 6077
Website: www.thebournetrust.org.uk
E-mail: info@thebournetrust.org.uk
Opening times: 9.00am–5.00pm, Mon–Thurs; 9.00am–4.00pm, Fri

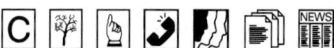

C 🌳 👆 📞 🦶 📑 NEWS

Description: The Bourne Trust provides professional counselling for remand prisoners. The Trust manages visitors' centres and play schemes at Wormwood Scrubs and Belmarsh Prisons. Volunteer groups visit prisoners at Holloway, Wakefield and Channings Wood.

Index keyword: General Information

Break

20 Hooks Hill Road
Sheringham
Norfolk
NR26 8NL

Admin tel: 01263 823170
Admin fax: 01263 825560
Website: www.break-charity.demon.co.uk
E-mail: office@break-charity.org

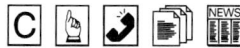

C 👆 📞 📑 NEWS

Description: BREAK provides a range of residential and day care services for children, adults and families with special needs, including holidays, respite care, child care and family assessments.

Index keyword: Disability: Care Scheme/Holidays

Breakthrough (Deaf/Hearing Integration)

Alan Geale House
West Hill Campus
The Close
Bristol Road
Selly Oak
Birmingham
B29 6LN

Admin tel: 0121 472 6447
Admin fax: 0121 415 2323
Website: www.breakthrough-DHI.org.uk

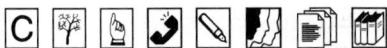

Description: Breakthrough is committed to integrating deaf and hearing people of all ages. Through contact, information and training.

Index keyword: Hearing Problems/ Deafness

Breast Cancer Care

Kiln House
210 New Kings Road
London
SW6 4NZ

Helpline tel: 0808 800 6000
Admin tel: 020 7384 2984
Admin fax: 020 7384 3387
Website: www.breastcancercare.org.uk
E-mail: bcc@breastcancercare.org.uk

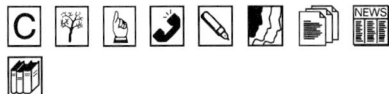

Description: Breat Cancer Care is the national organisation offering information and support to those affected by Breast Cancer. Our services are free, confidential and accessible.

Index keyword: Cancer

Breast Care Campaign

Blythe Hall
100 Blythe Road
London
W14 0HB

Admin tel: 020 7371 1510
Admin fax: 020 7371 4598

Description: The campaign was founded to promote education and information on non-cancerous breast disorders. A breast health resource pack for women and nurses is also available.

Index keyword: Women's Health

Brent Sickle Cell/Thalassaemia Centre

122 High Street
Harlesden
London
NW10 4SP

Admin tel: 020 8961 9005
Admin fax: 020 8453 0681

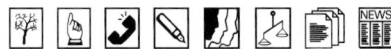

Description: Aims to promote awareness of sickle cell, thalassaemia and related conditions. Offers advice, information and support to people with these conditions. Free screening and counselling services for the general public, on a drop-in basis.

Index keyword: Sickle Cell/Thalassaemia

Bretforton Academy, The

Bretforton Hall
Main Street
Bretforton
Vale of Evesham
Worcestershire
WR11 5JH

Admin tel: 01386 830537
Admin fax: 01386 830918

Description: The Bretforton Academy conducts research into the treatment of various medical conditions including scleroderma and allied conditions.

Index keyword: General Information

British Acoustic Neuroma Association

Oak House
Ramsdon Wood Business Park
Southwell Road West
Mansfield
Nottinghamshire
NG21 0HJ

Admin tel: 01623 632143
Admin fax: 01623 635313
Website: www.ukan.co.uk/Bana
E-mail: bana@btclick.com

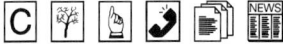

Description: The Association gives support, sympathetic listening and information interchange. Membership fee includes quarterly newsletter and invitation to open meetings with speakers. Also provides literature regarding Acoustic neuroma

Index keyword: General Information

British Acupuncture Council

63 Jeddo Road
London
W12 9HQ

Admin tel: 020 8735 0400
Admin fax: 020 8735 0404
Website: www.acupuncture.org.uk
E-mail: info@acupuncture.org.uk

Description: The British Acupuncture Council works to maintain common standards of education, ethics, discipline and codes of practice to ensure the health of the public at all times. It is committed to prompting research and enhancing the role that traditional acupuncture can play in the health and well being of the nation.

Index keyword: Complementary Medicine

British Agencies for Adoption and Fostering (BAAF)

Skyline House
200 Union Street
London
SE1 0LX

Admin tel: 020 7593 2000
Admin fax: 020 7593 2001
Website: www.baaf.org.uk
E-mail: mail@baaf.org.uk

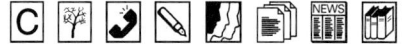

Description: Aims to improve the opportunities for family life for all children looked after by local authorities. Offers consultancy, training, publication and specialist family finding service.

Index keyword: Adoption and Fostering

British Allergy Foundation, The

Deepdene House
30 Bellegrove Road
Welling
Kent
DA16 3PY

Admin tel: 020 8303 8792
Admin fax: 020 7601 8444

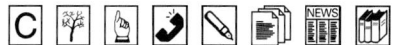

Description: The Foundation works to produce educational literature, to improve awareness of allergy, and to raise money for research.

Index keyword: Allergies

British Association for Counselling

1 Regent Place
Rugby
Warwickshire
CV21 2PJ

Helpline tel: 01788 578328

[C] [tree] [finger] [phone] [pencil] [pages] [NEWS] [book]

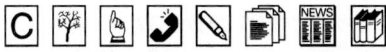

Description: Promotes understanding and awareness of counselling; aims to maintain and work towards raising standards of counselling, training and practice. Responds to requests for information and advice on matters related to counselling.

Index keyword: Counselling

British Association of Aesthetic Plastic Surgeons

The Royal College of Surgeons
35–43 Lincoln's Inn Fields
London
WC2A 3PN

Admin tel: 020 7405 2234
Admin fax: 020 7831 4041
Website: www.baaps.org.uk
E-mail: julia@baaps.org.uk

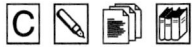

[C] [pencil] [pages] [book]

Description: Members of the public must specify procedure and enclose an sae.

Index keyword: Plastic Surgery

British Association of Cancer United Patients (BACUP)

3 Bath Place
Rivington Street
London
EC2A 3JR

Helpline tel: **0808 800 1234**
Admin tel: 020 7696 9003
Admin fax: 020 7696 9002
Opening times: 9am–7pm Mon–Fri

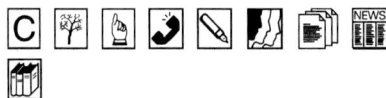

[C] [tree] [finger] [phone] [pencil] [leg] [pages] [NEWS]
[book]

Description: BACUP is the leading national charity providing information and support for people affected by cancer. All services are free of charge and confidential. Glasgow counselling: 0141 553 1553.

Index keyword: Cancer

British Association of Dermatologists

19 Fitzroy Square
London
W1P 6EH

Admin tel: 020 7383 0266
Admin fax: 020 7388 5263
Website: www.bad.org.uk
E-mail: admin@bad.org.uk

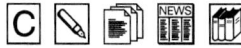

[C] [pencil] [pages] [NEWS] [book]

Description: Works to promote, for public benefit, greater knowledge and understanding of disease of the skin and to improve the teaching of dermatology at all levels, by organising and sponsoring scientific meetings, conferences and seminars; to stimulate and promote appropriate medical and scientific research.

Index keyword: Skin Problems

British Association of Homoepathic Veterinary Surgeons

Alternative Veterinary Medicine Centre
Chinham House
Stanford in the Vale
Oxon
SN7 8NQ

Admin tel: 01367 710324
Admin fax: 01367 718243

NEWS

Description: The Association promotes homoeopathic veterinary medicine and education and clinical research in homoeopathic veterinary medicine. It holds seminars, publishes newsletters for members and helps members of the public to locate veterinary help in homoeopathy.

Index keyword: General Information

British Association of Psychotherapists, The

37 Mapesbury Road
London
NW2 4HJ

Admin tel: 020 8452 9823
Admin fax: 020 8452 5182
Website: www.bat-psychotherapy.org
E-mail: mail@bat-psychotherapy.org

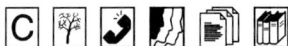

Description: Founded in 1951, this is one of the few professional bodies in the UK which has trained and qualified adult, adolescent and child analytic psychotherapists to a very high level of competence.

Index keyword: Psychotherapy

British Autogenic Society

Royal London Homeopathic Hospital
Great Ormond Street
London
WC1N 3HR

Admin tel: 020 7713 6636
Admin fax: 020 7713 6636
E-mail: autosoc@lineone.net

British Brain and Spine Foundation

35–43 Lincoln's Inn Fields
London
WC2A 3PN

Admin tel: 020 7404 6106
Admin fax: 020 7404 6105

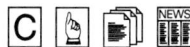

Description: By funding medical research and education programmes, the British Brain and Spine Foundation is working to improve our understanding and knowledge of disorders of the brain and spine throughout the medical world and general public alike.

Index keyword: Neurological

British Brain Tumour Association

2 Oakfield Road
Hightown
Merseyside
L38 9GQ

Helpline tel: 0151 929 3229
Admin tel: 0151 929 3229
Admin fax: 0151 929 3229

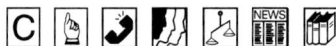

Description: To develop and set up local branches and support groups around the country. To promote public awareness and to raise funds for brain tumour research. To provide information to help patients and families who are suffering from this disease.

Index keyword: General Information

British Cardiac Patients Association, The (Zipper Club)

Unit 5d
2 Station Road
Swavesey
Cambridge
CB4 5QJ

Helpline tel: **01223 846845**
Admin tel: 01954 202022
Admin fax: 01954 202022 (fax/tel)
Website: www.easyweb.usernet.co.uk/bcpa
E-mail: bcpa@easynet.co.uk

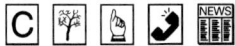

[C] [🌳] [✋] [📞] [NEWS]

Description: Offers help and support to all cardiac patients and their families, especially those awaiting heart surgery. Telephone helpline service. Run local support groups throughout the British Isles. Bi-monthly magazine.

Index keyword: Heart Problems

British Chiropractic Association

Blagrave House
17 Blagrave Street
Reading
Berks
RG1 1QB

Helpline tel: **0118 950 5950**
Admin tel: 01734 757557
Admin fax: 0118 958 8946

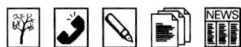

[🌳] [📞] [✏️] [📄] [NEWS]

Description: Promotes, encourages and maintains high standards of professional conduct, practice and educational training within the chiropractic profession. The BCA actively aims to increase awareness amongst the public and healthcare professions of chiropractic

as a safe and effective system of treatment for a variety of musculo-skeletal complaints.

Index keyword: Chiropractic

British Colostomy Association

15 Station Road
Reading
Berkshire
RG1 1LG

Helpline tel: **0800 328 4257**
Admin fax: 01189 569095
Opening times: Mon-Thurs 9am-3.30pm, Fri 9am-3pm

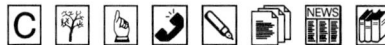

[C] [🌳] [✋] [📞] [✏️] [📄] [NEWS] [📖]

Description: Gives help, support and advice to anyone about to have/or who has a colostomy to return to a full and active life. They also have 25 area organisers throughout the country who also have a colostomy.

Index keyword: Digestive Problems

British Computer Society Disability Group, The

c/o West Hanningfield Road
Great Baddow
Chelmsford
CM2 8HN

Admin tel: 01245 242950
Admin fax: 01245 242924

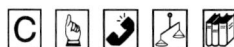

[C] [✋] [📞] [♿] [📖]

Description: Aims to demonstrate to employers and the public that IT is a tool for equality in the workplace. Represents to government the IT-related interests of disabled people and works with the computer industry to encourage producers of hardware and software to

31

consider disabled people at product design stage.

Index keyword: Disability: Equipment

British Council for Prevention of Blindness

12 Harcourt Street
London
W1H 1DS

Admin tel: 020 7724 3716
Admin fax: 020 7262 6199
E-mail: bcpb@globalnet.co.uk

Description: The aim of the BCPB is to fund medical research into preventing and treating blindness, both in the UK and the developing world. Grants are normally £10,000–£15,000 each for a maximum of three years.

Index keyword: Blindness/Visual Handicap

British Council of Organisations of Disabled People (BCODP)

Litchurch Plaza
Litchurch Lane
Derby
DE24 8AA

Info: **01332 298288**
Admin tel: 01332 295551
Admin fax: 01332 295580
Minicom: 01332 295581
Website: www.bcodp.org.uk
E-mail: bcodp@bcodp.org.uk
Opening times: 1.30pm–4.00pm

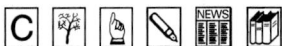

Description: BCODP is a national umbrella organisation representing 112 groups of disabled people. Since 1981, BCODP has campaigned for full civil

rights legislation for all disabled people. BCODP now offers an individual membership scheme.

Index keyword: Disability: General Information

British Deaf Association Health Promotion Unit

9 Springfield Street
Warrington
Cheshire
WA1 1BB

Helpline tel: **01925 652529**
Admin tel: 01925 652520
Admin fax: 01925 652526
Website: www.bda.org.uk
E-mail: bda6@dircon.co.uk
Opening times: 9.00am–4.30pm;
Wed, 1.00pm–10.00pm

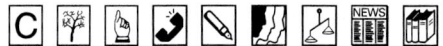

Description: The broad aims of the BDA are to advance and protect the interests of deaf people, develop pride, identify leadership qualities and awareness of their rights and responsibilities, thereby strengthening their own community and enabling them to take their place as full members of the wider national community. Provides health and sex education for any deaf or hard of hearing person, counselling in sign language, minicom counselling face-to-face and workshops. Aims to ensure that deaf and hard of hearing people have access to health issues.

Index keyword: Hearing Problems/Deafness

British Dental Health Foundation

Eastlands Court
St Peter's Road
Rugby
CV21 3QP

Admin tel: 01788 546365
Admin fax: 01788 541982
Website: www.dentalhouse.org.uk
Opening times: 9am–5pm, Mon–Fri

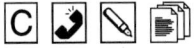

C ☎ ✎ 🗐

Description: Promotes the benefits of dental care to the general public and answers written enquiries on any aspect of dentistry.

Index keyword: Dental Health

British Dietetic Association

5th Floor, Elizabeth House
22 Suffolk Street, Queensway
Birmingham
West Midlands
B1 1LS

Admin tel: 0121 616 4900
Admin fax: 0121 616 4901
E-mail: info@bda.uk.com
Website: www.bda.uk.com

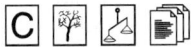

C 🌳 📐 🗐

Description: The British Dietetic Association provides training and communication facilities for State Registered Dieticians. The Association aims to inform, protect, represent and support its members. It publishes career information, manufactured food lists and policy documents.

Index keyword: Nutrition/Diet

British Digestive Foundation

3 St Andrews Place
London
NW1 4LB

Admin tel: 020 7486 0341
Admin fax: 020 7224 2012
Website: www.digestivedisorders.org.uk
E-mail: dds@digestivedisorders.org.uk

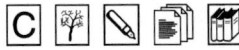

C 🌳 ✎ 🗐 📊

Description: The Foundation supports research and produces leaflets on common digestive disorders. These include indigestion, ulcers, heartburn, irritable bowel syndrome, gall-stones, constipation, diarrhoea, travellers' diarrhoea, maintaining bowel control, food poisoning and hepatitis. Enquirers should write to PO Box 251, Edgware, Middlesex, HA8 6HG, enclosing sae.

Index keyword: Digestive Problems

British DSP Support Group, The

Room 2
Monthamel House
Chapel Place
Ramsgate
Kent
CT11 9RY

Helpline tel: 01843 587356
Admin fax: 01843 587523
Website: www.dsp.future.easyspace.com
E-mail: britishdspsupport@compuserve.com

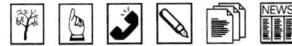

🌳 👆 ☎ ✎ 🗐 NEWS

Description: The Group aims to put sufferers from DSP in touch with one another and disseminate information gathered by members, branches, professional and medical bodies; to bring this under-diagnosed condition to the attention of the medical profession; to investigate the causes; to get DSP recognised as a disability.

Index keyword: General Information

British Dyslexia Association

98 London Road
Reading
Berkshire
RG1 5AU

Helpline tel: 0118 966 8277
Admin tel: 0118 966 2677
Admin fax: 0118 935 1927

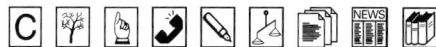

Description: The BDA represents over two million children and adults with dyslexia. They believe that difficulties can be significantly reduced by early intervention, suitable teaching methods and helpful learning skills.

Index keyword: Dyslexia

British Epilepsy Association

New Anstey House
Gateway Drive
Yeadon
Leeds
LS19 7XY
Helpline tel: 0808 800 5050
Admin tel: 0113 210 8800
Admin fax: 0113 391 0300
Website: www.epilepsy.org.uk
E-mail: epilepsy@bea.org.uk
Opening times: 9.00am–4.30pm, Mon–Thurs; 9.00am–4.00pm, Fri

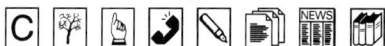

Description: Provides video packages for education and training and organises seminars. Epdata is a medical literature search service: tel. 0113 2108 851

Index keyword: Epilepsy

British Fluoridation Society

4th Floor
University of Liverpool School of Dentistry
Liverpool
L69 3BX

Helpline tel: 0151 706 5216
Admin tel: 0151 706 5216
Admin fax: 0151 706 5845

Description: Aims to improve oral health by securing the optimum fluoride content of water.

Index keyword: General Information

British Heart Foundation

14 Fitzhardinge Street
London
W1H 4DH

Heart Health line: 0870 600 6566
Admin tel: 020 7487 7178
Admin fax: 020 7486 5820
Website: www.bhf.org.uk
Opening times: 24 hours

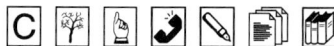

Index keyword: Heart Problems

British Herbal Medicine Association

Sun House
Church Street
Stroud
Gloucestershire
GL5 1SL

Helpline tel: 01453 751389
Admin tel: 01453 751389
Admin fax: 01453 751402

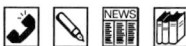

Description: The Association aims to defend the right of the public to choose herbal remedies and to be able to obtain them freely; to encourage wider knowledge and recognition of the value of herbal medicine; to promote high standards of quality and safety in herbal remedies. Newsletter provided for members.

Index keyword: Complementary Medicine

British Holistic Medical Association (BHMA)

Rowland Thomas House
Royal Shrewsbury Hospital South
Shrewsbury
SY3 8XF

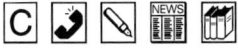

C ☎ ✎ NEWS 📖

Description: Holistic practitioners aim to treat patients as whole people with psychological, spiritual, emotional and social, as well as physical, needs. They believe this approach gives better healthcare and can help people towards self-healing. 'Holistic medicine' can include any form of healthcare, from major surgery to the laying on of hands, as long as it is practised according to these principles.

Index keyword: Complementary Medicine

British Homoeopathic Association

27a Devonshire Street
London
W1N 1RJ

Helpline tel: **020 7935 2163**

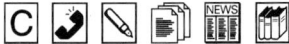

C ☎ ✎ 📄 NEWS 📖

Description: The association was founded in 1902 and aims to promote homoeopathy by all available means. Provides an information service, distributing lists of doctors and veterinary surgeons trained in homoeopathy. Maintains a library on premises for the use of members.

Index keyword: Complementary Medicine

British Homoeopathic Dental Association, The

2b Franklin Road
Watford
WD1 1QD

Helpline tel: **01923 233336**
Admin tel: 01923 233336

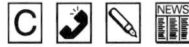

C ☎ ✎ NEWS

Description: Involved in the education of dentists in homoeopathic dentistry, dissemination and collation of available research and information. Provides the public with information on homoeopathic dentistry.

Index keyword: Dental Health

British Humanist Association

47 Theobalds Road
London
WC1X 8SP

Admin tel: 020 7430 0908
Admin fax: 020 7430 1271
Website: www.humanism.org.uk
E-mail: info@humansim.org.uk

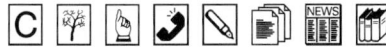

C 🌳 👆 ☎ ✎ 📄 NEWS 📖

Description: The BHA provides help, including hospital visiting and services for the non-religious; plus books on non-religious weddings, namings and funerals.

Index keyword: General Information

British Hypnotherapy Association

67 Upper Berkeley Street
London
W1H 7QX

Admin tel: 020 7723 4443

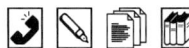

☎ ✎ 📄 📖

Description: This is a professional organisation of psychotherapists with at least four years of training in helping people to understand and resolve their emotional problems, relationship difficulties, neurotic behaviour, anxieties, migraine etc. Also sends literature regarding local practitioners and frequently asked questions.

Index keyword: Complementary Medicine

British Institute for Brain Injured Children, The

Knowle Hall
Knowle
Bridgewater
Somerset
TA7 8PJ

Admin tel: 01278 684060
Admin fax: 01278 685573

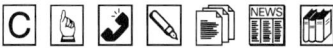

Description: BIBIC offers a fighting alternative to simply accepting brain injury as untreatable. Provides programmes of home stimulation therapy. These are taught to parents during a week of assessment and teaching and thereafter carried out at home by the parents and volunteer helpers to promote neurological development. Four-monthly reassessments enable adjustments to treatment techniques, as necessary.

Index keyword: Neurological

British Institute of Learning Disabilities

Wolverhampton Road
Kidderminster
Worcestershire
DY10 3PP

Admin tel: 01562 850251
Admin fax: 01562 851970

Index keyword: Learning Disabilities

British Kidney Patient Association

Bordon
Hampshire
GU35 9JZ

Admin tel: 01420 472021; 01420 472022
Admin fax: 01420 475 831

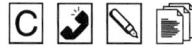

Description: To provide for the material and physical needs of kidney patients and families, to lobby for more and improved facilities, and increased government funding, so that all patients may benefit from improvements in technology and pharmaceutical achievements. Also to create awareness through the media of the need for kidney donors.

Index keyword: Kidney Disease

British Limbless Ex Servicemen's Association (BLESMA)

Franklin Moore House
185–187 High Road
Chadwell Heath
Essex
RM6 6NA

Admin tel: 020 8590 1124
Admin fax: 020 8599 2932
Website: www.blesma.org
E-mail: blesma@btconnect.com

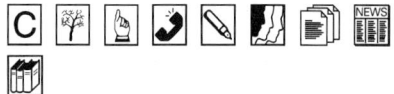

Description: Works for the welfare and well-being of serving and ex-service amputees, widows and families. Grants, rehabilitation, residential and nursing homes. Advice on pensions and allowances. Consumer watchdog for artificial limbs and appliances.

Index keyword: Amputees

British Liver Trust

Ransomes Europark
Ipswich
IP3 9QG

Helpline tel: 0808 800 1000
Admin tel: 01473 276326
Admin fax: 01473 276327
Website: www.britishlivertrust.org.uk
E-mail: info@britishlivertrust.org.uk
Opening times: Weekdays 9.00am–5.00pm.

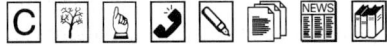

Description: Offers help and support to all adults suffering from liver disease.

Index keyword: Liver Disease

British Lung Foundation (Breathe Easy Club)

78 Hatton Garden
London
EC1N 8LD

Admin tel: 020 7831 5831
Admin fax: 020 7831 5832
Website: www.lunguk.org.uk
E-mail: blf-user@gpiag-asthma.org.uk

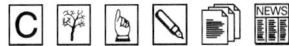

Description: The British Lung Foundation exists to fund research into all lung diseases, to provide public information on lung diseases and good lung health, and to support people with a lung condition through the Breathe Easy Club.

Index keyword: Lung Disease

British Medical Acupuncture Society

12 Marbury House
Higher Whitley
Warrington
Cheshire
WA4 4QW

Admin tel: 01925 730727
Admin fax: 01925 730492
Website: www.medical-acupuncture.co.uk
E-mail: bmasadmin@aol.com

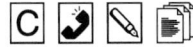

Description: Provides area lists of medical practitioners practising acupuncture and a patient advice leaflet.

Index keyword: Acupuncture

British Migraine Association

178a High Road
Byfleet
West Byfleet
Surrey
KT14 7ED

Helpline tel: 01932 352468
Admin fax: 01932 351257
Website: www.migraine.org.uk
E-mail: info@migraine.org.uk

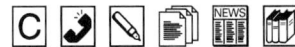

Description: Since 1958 the association has promoted and supported research into the cause and treatment of migraine. Provides encouragement and information to enable many sufferers from migraine to control their attacks and live normal lives.

Index keyword: Migraine

British Nutrition Foundation, The

High Holborn House
52–54 High Holborn
London
WC1V 6RQ

Admin tel: 020 7404 6504
Admin fax: 020 7404 6747
Website: www.nutrition.org.uk
E-mail: postbox@nutrition.org.uk

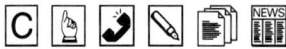

Description: The British Nutrition Foundation was established as an impartial scientific charity, providing reliable information and scientifically-based advice on nutrition and related health matters. The ultimate objective of the Foundation is to help consumers to understand the relationship between nutrition, diet and lifestyle.

Index keyword: Nutrition/Diet

British Organisation of Non-parents (BON)

BM Box 5866
London
WC1N 3XX

Admin tel: 01923 856177

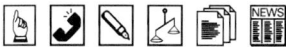

Description: Promotes the views of those who choose not to have children and a positive view of the child-free life. Offers support, advice and solidarity to people under pressure or having difficulty deciding and believes firmly that parenthood should be seen as an option, not a duty or a necessity.

Index keyword: General Information

British Pensioners and Trade Union Action Association

Norman Dodds House
315 Bexley Road
Erith
Kent
DA8 3EX

Admin tel: 01322 335464
Admin fax: 01322 335464

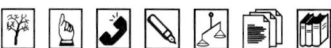

Description: Aims to campaign on the many issues concerning pensioners and to improve their standard of living.

Index keyword: Elderly: General Information

British Polio Fellowship

Ground Floor, Unit a
Eagle Office Centre, The Runway
South Ruislip
Middlesex
HA4 6SE

Helpline tel: **0800 0180 586**
Admin tel: 020 8842 1898
Admin fax: 020 8842 0555
Website: under construction
E-mail: british.polio@dial.pipex.com
Opening times: 8.00am–5.00pm

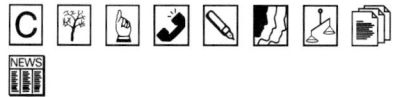

Description: Grants for polio-disabled people resident in the UK. Accessible holiday accommodation. Twenty-bed residential care home for polio-disabled people.

Index keyword: Polio

British Pregnancy Advisory Service

Austy Manor
Wootton Wawen
Solihull
West Midlands
B95 6BX

Helpline tel: **08457 304030**
Admin tel: 01564 793225
Admin fax: 01564 794935

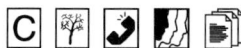

Description: BPAS is a charity-based organisation with branches throughout the country, offering information, counselling and treatment in a range of services linked with fertility controls and unplanned pregnancy.

Index keyword: Pregnancy and Childbirth

British Psychological Society

48 Princess Road East
Leicester
LE1 7DR

Admin tel: 0116 254 9568
Admin fax: 0116 247 0787
Website: www.bps.org.uk
E-mail: mail@bps.org

C 🌳 📖

Description: If a client wishes to consult with a psychologist, they should either use referral services of a GP or consult the *Directory of Chartered Psychologists*, available in main reference libraries.

Index keyword: Psychology

British Red Cross

9 Grosvenor Crescent
London
SW1X 7EJ

Admin tel: 020 7235 5454
Admin fax: 020 7245 6315
Website: www.redcross.org.uk
E-mail: information@redcross.org.uk

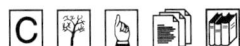

C 🌳 ✋ 📄 📖

Description: The British Red Cross cares for people in crisis everywhere – meeting the needs of vulnerable people in times of emergency.

Index keyword: General Information

British Reflexology Association

Monks Orchard
Whitbourne
Worcester
Worcestershire
WR6 5RB

Admin tel: 01886 821207
Admin fax: 01886 822017
Website: www.britreflex.co.uk
E-mail: bra@britflex.co.uk

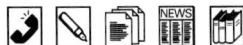

📞 ✏️ 📄 NEWS 📖

Description: Professional body representing reflexology practitioners aiming to promote its members and the method of reflexology in general.

Index keyword: Complementary Medicine

British Retinitis Pigmentosa Society

PO Box 350
Buckingham
MK18 5EL

Helpline tel: **01280 860363**
Admin tel: 01280 860195
Admin fax: 01280 860515
Website: www.brps.demon.co.uk
E-mail: lynda@brps.demon.co.uk
Opening times: 9am–10pm.

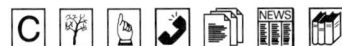

C 🌳 ✋ 📞 📄 NEWS 📖

Description: BRPS gives people the opportunity to meet fellow-sufferers and resolve common problems. It works towards the common goal of finding a cure.

Index keyword: Blindness/Visual Handicap

British School of Experimental and Clinical Hypnosis

Psychology Consultancy
District General Hospital, Scartho Road
Scarth Road
Grimsby
DN33 2BA

Admin tel: 01472 873423
Opening times: 8.30am–7pm

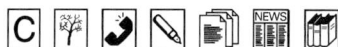

Description: Promotes the scientific study of hypnosis, appreciates clinical use and provides information and assistance to professionals and members of the public. Newsletter is produced for members only.

Index keyword: Hypnosis

British School of Osteopathy, The

275 Borough High Street
London
SE1 1JE

Clinic helpline: **020 7407 0222**
School: 020 7407 0222
Admin fax: 020 7839 1098
Website: www.bfo.ac.uk
E-mail: admin@bfo.ac.uk

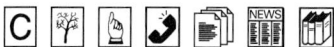

Description: Promotes osteopathy and its contribution to the provision of contemporary health care.

Index keyword: Holistic

British School of Reflexology

92 Sheering Road
Old Harlow
Essex
CM17 0JW

Helpline tel: **01279 429060**
Admin fax: 01279 445234
E-mail: reflexology.brf@tesco.net
Opening times: 9.00am–5.30pm

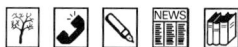

Description: The British School of Reflexology offers training in reflexology; treatment; and mail order catalogues giving a variety of books, charts, treatment couches and chairs for the reflexologist.

Index keyword: Holistic

British Sjögrens Syndrome Association

20 Kingston Way
Nailsea
Bristol
BS19 2RA

Helpline tel: **01275 854215**
Admin tel: 01275 854215

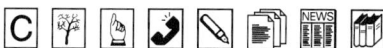

Description: Aims to help patients and their families understand and cope better with the disease. Also tries to make medical professionals more aware of patients' problems.

Index keyword: Sjögrens Syndrome

British Ski Club for the Disabled

Springmount
Berwick St John
Shaftesbury
Dorset
SP7 0HQ

Helpline tel: **01784 431234**
Admin tel: 01784 431234

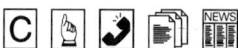

Description: Trains guides to assist skiers with various disabilities; provides and develops specialist skiing aids and equipment; offers ski guiding and practice sessions on artificial slopes; organises snow holidays for groups.

Index keyword: Disability: Sport/Exercise

British Snoring and Sleep Apnoea Association, The (BSSAA)

How Lane
Chipstead
Surrey
CR5 3LT

Helpline tel: **01249 557997**
Admin tel: 01249 701010
Admin fax: 01737 248744
Opening times: 9am–9pm
E-mail: marianne@britishsnoring.co.uk

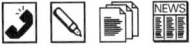

Description: Provides information on causes, advises on remedies, gives help and support to people affected by snoring and sleep apnoea. Anti-snoring and apnoea prevention devices available.

Index keyword: Sleep Problems

British Society for Allergy and Environmental Medicine

PO Box 28
Totton
Southampton
SO40 2ZA

Admin tel: 023 8081 2124
Admin tel: 023 8081 3912

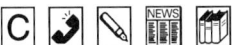

Description: British Society for Allergy and Environmental Medicine with British Society for Nutritional Medicine encourages the use of environmental and nutritional medicine to prevent symptoms, rather than suppress them with drugs. This is a society of medical practitioners and scientific members. Patients are seen only on referral by their GPs.

Index keyword: Allergies

British Society for Music Therapy

25 Rosslyn Avenue
East Barnet
Hertfordshire
EN4 8DH

Helpline tel: **020 8368 8879**
Admin fax: 020 8368 8879

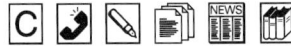

Description: Promotes music therapy. Holds meetings and conferences. Publishes a journal and bulletin for members. Sells books and videos.

Index keyword: Music

British Stammering Association, The

15 Old Ford Road
London
E2 9PJ

Helpline tel: **0845 603 2001**
Admin tel: 020 8983 1003
Admin fax: 020 8983 3591
Website: www.stammering.org
E-mail: mail@stammering.org

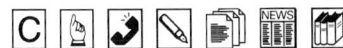

Description: Helps people of all ages who stammer, to communicate more effectively. Produces literature for people of all ages who stammer.

Index keyword: Speech Difficulties

British Thyroid Foundation

PO Box 97
Clifford
Wetherby
West Yorkshire
LS23 6XD

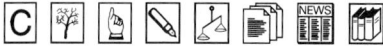

C 🌳 ✋ ✏️ 🔬 🗐 NEWS 📖

Description: Provides support and clear information to sufferers of thyroid disorders; promotes greater awareness of these disorders among the general public and medical profession; helps set up regional support groups; and raises funds for research.

Index keyword: Thyroid

British Tinnitus Association

4th Floor
White Building
FitzAllen Square
Sheffield
S1 2AZ

Helpline tel: 0800 0180527
Admin tel: 0114 279 6600
Admin fax: 0114 279 6222
Website: www.tinnitus.org.uk
E-mail: bta@tinnitus.org.uk

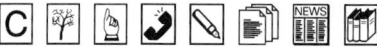

C 🌳 ✋ 📞 ✏️ 🗐 NEWS 📖

Description: Provides information, help and support for people with tinnitus and other interested parties. Aims to promote awareness and encourage formation of self-help groups.

Index keyword: Hearing Problems/ Deafness

British Wheel of Yoga

1 Hamilton Place
Boston Road
Sleaford
Lincolnshire
NG34 7ES

Admin tel: 01529 306851
Admin fax: 01529 303233
Website: www.bwy.org.uk
E-mail: wheelyoga@aol.com

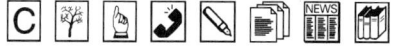

C 🌳 ✋ 📞 ✏️ 🗐 NEWS 📖

Description: Encourages and helps people to a greater knowledge and understanding of all aspects of yoga and its practice, by the provision of study, education and training. Activities include seminars, teacher training, in-service training, regional and national AGMs, annual congress, national training week and diploma course tutor training weekend.

Index keyword: Complementary Medicine

British Wireless for the Blind Fund

Gabriel House
34 New Road
Chatham
Kent
ME4 4QR

Admin tel: 01634 832501
Admin fax: 01634 817485
Website: www.blind.org.uk
E-mail: margeret@blind.org.uk

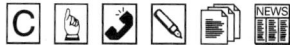

C ✋ 📞 ✏️ 🗐 NEWS

Description: The Fund provides radios/radio cassette players on a free permanent loan basis to the registered blind in need.

Index keyword: Blindness/Visual Handicap

Brittle Bone Society

30 Guthrie Street
Dundee
DD1 5BS

Helpline tel: **0800 0282459**
Admin tel: 01382 204446
Admin fax: 01382 206771
Website: www.brittlebone.org
E-mail: bbs@brittlebone.org
Opening times: 9.00am–4.30pm

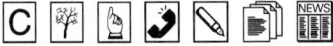

[icons]

Description: The Society seeks to promote research into the causes, inheritance and treatment of osteogenesis imperfecta and similar disorders characterised by excessive fragility of the bones. It also provides advice, encouragement and practical help for patients and their relatives facing the difficulties of living with brittle bones.

Index keyword: Brittle Bone Diseases

Brook Advisory Centres

421 Highgate Studios
53–79 Highgate Road
London
NW5 1TL

Helpline tel: **08000 185 023**
Admin tel: 020 7284 6040
Admin fax: 020 7284 6050
E-mail: information@brookcentres.org.uk
Opening times: 9.00am–5.00pm,
Mon–Thurs; 9.00am–4.00pm, Fri

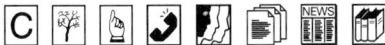

[icons]

Description: Brook Centres offer young people free, confidential contraceptive advice and supplies, and help with emotional and sexual problems. There are 35 centres throughout the country, visited by over 66,000 young men and women each year.

Index keyword: Sexual Problems

C

Calibre

Aylesbury
Buckinghamshire
HP22 5XQ

Helpline tel: **01296 432339**
Admin tel: 01296 432339
Admin fax: 01296 392599

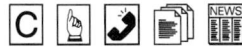

[icons]

Description: Calibre provides a free library service of unabridged books on cassette for the blind and print-disabled. The cassettes are available for people of all ages and can be played on standard equipment.

Index keyword: Blindness/Visual Handicap

Calvert Trust Keswick, The

Little Crosthwaite
Keswick
Cumbria
CA12 4QD

Admin tel: 01768 772254
Admin fax: 017687 771298
Website: www.calvert-trust.org.uk
E-mail: calvert.keswick@dial.pipex.com

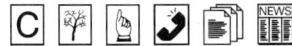

[icons]

Description: The Calvert Trust aims to enable people with any kind of physical, sensory or mental disability to benefit from outdoor activities in the countryside, by the provision of access to such activities, safe and competent instruction and appropriate accommodation.

Index keyword: Disability: Care Scheme/Holidays

Campaign for Homosexual Equality

PO Box 342
London
WC1X ODU

Admin tel: 0770 2326151
Admin fax: 020 8743 6252

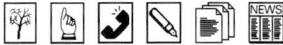

Description: CHE is a voluntary organisation working to change attitudes and laws that make life difficult for homosexual and bisexual people.

Index keyword: Gays/Lesbians

Camphill Village Trust

19 South Road
Stourbridge
West Midlands
DY8 3YA

Helpline tel: 01384 441505 Mornings 9.30–12.30 pm

Admin tel: 01384 372122
Admin fax: 01384 372122
Website: www.camphill.org.uk

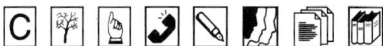

Description: The trust consists of communities including people with special needs, in urban and rural settings; opportunities are given for work, social and cultural activities.

Index keyword: Mental Health/Illness

Cancer and Leukaemia In Childhood (CLIC)

Abbey Wood
Bristol
BS34 7JU

Helpline tel: **0117 3112600**
Admin fax: 0117 3112694

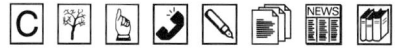

Description: CLIC aims to help children suffering from cancer and leukaemia and their parents. This help covers an all-embracing range of services, such as welfare grants, research and treatment. CLIC receives no government money at all and relies entirely on voluntary donations to fund its services.

Index keyword: Cancer

Cancer Bacup

3 Bath Place
Rivington Street
London
EC2A 3JR

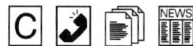

Helpline: **0808 800 1234**
Admin tel: 020 7696 9003
Admin fax: 020 7696 9002
Website: www.cancerbacup.org.uk
E-mail: info@cancerbacup.org.uk
Opening times: 9.00am–7.00pm; Mon–Fri

Description: Cancer Bacup is the leading national charity providing information and support for people affected by cancer. All services are free and confidential.

Cancer Care Society

11 The Corn Market
Romsey
Hampshire
SO51 8GB

Admin tel: 01794 830300
Admin fax: 01794 518133
Website: www.cancercaresoc.demon.co.uk
E-mail: info@cancercaresoc.demon.co.uk

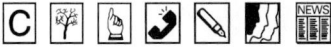

Description: The society provides free and confidential information, a counselling centre, support groups, complementary therapies, wig-fitting service and holiday accommodation.

Index keyword: Cancer

Cancer Laryngectomee Trust

Claremount House
Claremount Road
Halifax
HX3 6AW

Helpline tel: 01422 844992

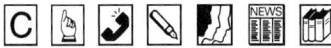

Description: The charity provides support for neck breathers and their families, and liaison with speech therapists. Aims to raise awareness of speech disability.

Index keyword: Cancer

Cancer Research Campaign

10 Cambridge Terrace
London
NW1 4JL

Helpline: 0800 226237
Admin tel: 020 7224 1333
Admin fax: 020 7487 4310
Website: www.crc.org.uk
E-mail: crcinformation@crc.org.uk

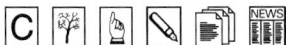

Description: Is Britain's leading cancer charity and funds around ⅓ of all research into cancer in UK. Is European leader into anti-cancer drug development.

Cancer You Are Not Alone (CYANA)

31 Church Road
Manor Park
London
E12 6AD

Admin tel: 020 8553 5366
Admin fax: 020 8553 5366

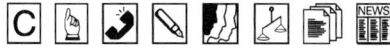

Description: CYANA is a Newham-based cancer self-help group for anyone with a cancer-related problem, whether they are the patient, relative, carer or friend and regardless of age, creed, nationality or lifestyle. The charity provides counselling, weekly drop-in meetings (Tues/Wed), information, help and advice. Also provides an Asian Link worker.

Index keyword: Cancer

Cancerkin

Royal Free Hospital
Hampstead
London
NW3 2QG

Admin tel: 020 7830 2323
Admin fax: 020 7830 2324

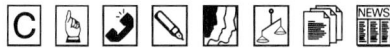

Description: Offers supportive care and rehabilitation, extra to the NHS, for people with breast cancer. Also provides education and training for health professionals and lay volunteers; public and professional information; fund-raising to support all programmes.

Index keyword: Cancer

Cancerlink

17 Britannia Street
London
WC1X 9JN

Helpline tel: **020 7833 2451; 0800 132905**
Admin tel: 020 7833 2818
Admin fax: 020 7833 4963

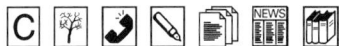

Description: Provides emotional support and information on all aspects of cancer in response to letter and telephone enquiries from people with cancer, their families, friends and professionals working with them. Acts as a resource for over 500 cancer support and self-help groups throughout the UK.

Index keyword: Cancer

Canine Partners for Independence

Homewell House
22 Homewell
Havant
Hampshire
PO9 1EE

Admin tel: 02392 450156
Admin fax: 02392 470140
Website: www.cpiuk.org

E-mail: cpi@cpiuk.org

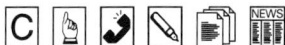

Description: Provides trained dogs to assist severely physically disabled people with the tasks of every day life and thus enabling them achieve greater independence.

Index keyword: Disability: General Information

Cara Trust, The

178 Lancaster Road
London
W11 1QU

Admin tel: 020 7792 8299
Admin fax: 020 7792 8004
E-mail: lindsay@caratrust.freeserve.co.uk

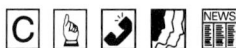

Description: Cara (A community of friendly people living with HIV) provides one-to-one pastoral/emotional/spiritual support, bereavement support, funeral planning and taking, support groups, hospital/home support, complementary therapies, drop-in services and women's Wednesdays.

Index keyword: AIDS and HIV

Cardiomyopathy Association

40 The Metro Centre
Tolpits Lane
Watford
Hertfordshire
WD1 8SB

Admin tel: 01923 249977
Admin fax: 01923 249987
Website: www.cardiomyopathy.org
E-mail: cmaassoc@aol.com

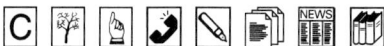

Description: To help alleviate concern among potential and diagnosed sufferers; their families; advisors; and the media, by giving support and assistance in an empathetic but professional manner.

Care Alternatives

206 Worple Road
Wimbledon
London
SW20 8AZ

Helpline tel: **020 8946 8202**
Admin tel: 020 8946 8202
Admin fax: 020 8944 7431

Description: Care workers are available to assist people in their own homes, on a flexible basis, from one hour right up to live-in help. The service is managed by area managers (mainly nurses), who will visit to discuss needs and advise.

Index keyword: Disability: Care Scheme/Holidays

Care And Action Trust for Children with Handicaps, The (CATCH)

Oystermouth House
Charter Court
Phoenix Way, Enterprise Park
Swansea
SA7 9FS

Admin tel: 01792 790077
Admin fax: 01792 772137
Website: www.catchtrust.org.uk
E-mail: mail@catchtrust.org.uk

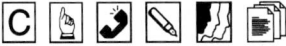

C 👆 📞 ✏️ 🦵 📄

Description: Provides practical assistance, guidance and counselling for families with a handicapped child. Promotes greater understanding, acceptance and integration of handicapped children. Collects and disseminates information on all issues relating to the handicap. Influences legislation affecting the disabled.

Index keyword: Disability: Children

Care of Next Infant (CONI)

Room CI, Stephenson Wing
Sheffield Children's Hospital
University of Sheffield, Western Bank
Sheffield
S10 2TH

Admin tel: 0114 276 6452
Website: www.sids.org.uk/FSID
E-mail: coni@sheffield.ac.uk

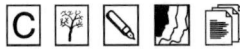

C 🌳 ✏️ 🦵 📄

Description: CONI is a programme used by hospitals and community health services to develop a system of practical help and professional support for every family with their subsequent babies after a cot death. Support available includes weekly visits by a health visitor, symptom diaries, apnoea monitor, weighing scales, weight chart and room thermometer.

Index keyword: Cot Death

Caring and Sharing Trust

Cotton's Farmhouse
Whiston Road
Cogenhoe
Northamptonshire
NN7 1NL

Admin tel: 01604 891487
Admin fax: 01604 890405

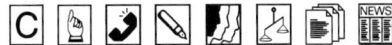

C 👆 📞 ✏️ 🦵 📐 📄 NEWS

Description: Provides opportunities and instruction for people with learning difficulties via day centre based arts and drama. There is a small residential section. Two seasons of shows a year in their own theatre by and for people with learning difficulties. Counselling advice and support for clients, their carers and professionals.

Index keyword: Mental Health/Illness

Caroline Flint Midwifery Services

34 Elm Quay Court
Nine Elms Lane
London
SW8 5DE

Admin tel: 020 7498 2322
Admin fax: 020 7498 0698
Website: www.birthcentre.com
E-mail: midwifecf@aol.com

[icons: telephone, documents]

Description: This is a group practice of independent midwives, providing women with antenatal care in their homes or in their offices at times convenient to them. They can deliver babies at home, in hospital or in their birth centre and provides advice and support to women, whatever form of childbirth they choose.

Index keyword: Pregnancy and Childbirth

Catholic Child Welfare Council

St Josephs
Walford Way
Hendon
London
NW4 4TY

Admin tel: 020 8203 6323
Admin fax: 020 8203 6323

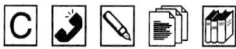

[icons: C, telephone, pencil, documents, book]

Description: A federation of Catholic caring agencies, Catholic children's societies and some religious congregations providing social care services for children and families in need. Promotes the care and welfare of children and families, co-ordinates resources, provides advice and training and ensures the maintenance of standards of professional practice.

Index keyword: Childcare

Catholic Deaf Association

Hensey House
Sudell Street
Collyhurst
Monchester
M4 4JG

Admin tel: 0161 8348828

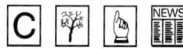

[icons: C, tree, hand, NEWS]

Description: Promotes, supports and helps develop services for deaf people in the Roman Catholic dioceses of Britain. Each diocese has its own local service for deaf people.

Index keyword: Hearing Problems/ Deafness

Central Council for Jewish Community Services

17 Highfield Road
Golders Green
London
NW11 9LS

Admin tel: 020 8458 1035
Admin fax: 020 8731 7462

[icons: C, documents, NEWS]

Description: The council unites the work of more than 60 Jewish community service organisations throughout the country. Services include: ombudsman; arbitration and mediation; Jewish emergency support service (for disasters); leadership courses; publication of the directory of Jewish social services; conferences; Jewish housing associations.

Index keyword: Ethnic Minorities

Centre for Accessible Environments

Nutmeg House
60 Gainsford Street
London
SE1 2NY

Admin tel: 020 7357 8182
Admin fax: 020 7357 8183
Website: www.cae.org.uk
E-mail: info@cae.org.uk

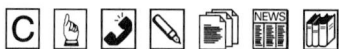

[icons: C, hand, telephone, pencil, documents, NEWS, book]

Description: CAE is a registered charity which provides information, training and consultancy on the design and adaptation of buildings and spaces to ensure that they are accessible to everyone including disabled and older people. Publishes design guides, provides in-house training, and carries out access appraisal of architects' drawings and access audits of buildings.

Index keyword: Disability: General Information

Centre for Brain Injury Rehabilitation and Development

131 Main Road
Broughton
Chester
CH4 0NR

Admin tel: 01244 532047
Admin fax: 01244 538723

C ✋ ✆ 🗐

Description: This is an outpatient clinic for children/adults suffering from congenital or traumatic brain injury, non-progressive. Patients are taken for one year, during which technical and subjective improvements have to occur. Specific movement patterns to inhibit primitive postural reflexes are done daily in patients' own homes.

Index keyword: Neurological

Centre for Complementary Health Studies

University of Exeter
Amory Building
Rennes Drive
Exeter
EX4 4RJ

Admin tel: 01392 264498
Admin fax: 01392 433828
Website: www.ex.ac/chs
E-mail: chs@ex.ac.uk

C

Description: A university department that offers postgraduate degrees in Complementary Health Studies and undertakes research in the field.

Index keyword: Holistic

Centre for Pregnancy Nutrition

The University of Sheffield
Clinical Sciences Centre
Northern General Hospital
Sheffield
S5 7AU

Helpline tel: **0114 242 4084**
Admin tel: 0114 271 4888
Admin fax: 0114 261 7584
E-mail: pregnancynutrition@shef.ac.uk
Opening times: 9.00am–4.00pm, Mon–Fri

✆ ✎ 🗐

Description: The eating for pregnancy helpline provides a service to members of the public, the media, fellow scientists and health professionals about nutrition before and during pregnancy and lactation.

Index keyword: Pregnancy and Childbirth

Cerebral Palsy Helpline (SCOPE)

PO Box 833
Milton Keynes
MK12 5NY

Helpline tel: **0808 800 3333**
Admin tel: 01908 321047
Admin fax: 01908 321051
Website: www.scope.org.uk
E-mail: cphelpline@scope.org.uk
Opening hours: 9.00am–9.00pm,
Weekdays; 2.00pm–6.00pm, Weekends

C

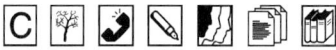

Description: The Cerebral Palsy Helpline is the national information and support line for SCOPE. It offers information, support and advice on cerebral palsy and associated disability disabilities and acts as a front line service for enquiries about SCOPE and its services.

Index keyword: Cerebral Palsy

Chai-Lifeline

Norwood House
Harmony Way
London
NW4 2BZ

Helpline tel: 0808 808 4567
Admin tel: 020 8202 2211
Admin fax: 020 8202 2111
E-mail: info@chai-lifeline.org.uk

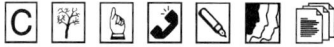

Description: Gives reassurance, support and friendship to Jewish cancer patients and their families. 24 hour helpline; weekly support meetings; general information service; home, hospital and hospice visiting; spiritual guidance; public lectures. Provides daily complementary therapy clinics, together with well woman and well man screening clinics.

Index keyword: Cancer

Charities Aid Foundation

Kings Hill
West Malling
Kent
ME19 4TA

Admin tel: 01732 520000
Admin fax: 01732 520001
Website: www.cafonline.org
E-mail: info@caf.charitynet.org
Website: www.caf.org

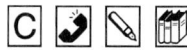

Description: Advises on sources of financial help; produces a guide to grant-making trusts; runs a give-as-you earn scheme.

Index keyword: General Information

Charity Search

25 Portview Road
Avonmouth
Bristol
BS11 9LD

Admin tel: 0117 982 4060
Admin fax: 0117 982 2846

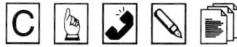

Description: Links elderly people in genuine financial difficulty with established charities that might help them. An experienced team responds promptly and sympathetically to enquiries, either by letter or telephone.

Index keyword: Elderly: General Information

Chest Heart and Stroke Scotland

65 North Castle Street
Edinburgh
EH2 3LT

Helpline tel: 01845 0776000
Admin tel: 0131 225 6963
Admin fax: 0131 220 6313
Opening times: 9:30am–4pm, Weekdays

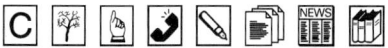

Description: This medical charity aims to improve the quality of life for people affected by chest, heart and stroke illness, through research, health education advice and information and provision of services.

Index keyword: Stroke

Child

Charter House
43 St Leonards Road
Bexhill on Sea
East Sussex
TN40 1JA

Admin tel: 01424 732361
Admin fax: 01424 731858
Website: www.child.org.uk
E-mail: office@email2.child.org.uk

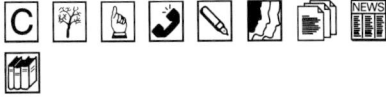

[icons]

Description: Provides high quality support, helplines and information to people suffering the effects of infertility. Promotes public awareness and encourages mutual support.

Index keyword: Infertility

Child Accident Prevention Trust

Clerks Court
18–20 Farringdon Lane
London
EC1R 3HA

Admin tel: 020 7608 3828
Admin fax: 020 7608 3674
E-mail: safe@capt.demon.co.uk

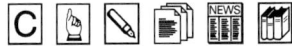

[icons]

Description: The Trust works to reduce the number and severity of preventable childhood accidents in the UK, through information, research and national campaigns, such as child safety week (run annually).

Index keyword: Accident Prevention

Child and Family Trust

Fleming House
134 Renfrew Street
Glasgow
G3 6ST

Admin tel: 0141 353 2424
Admin fax: 0141 353 3435
Website: www.cft-scotland.com
E-mail: info@cft-scotland.com

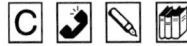

[icons]

Description: Support Fulton MacKay Nurse Projects to help children and families with emotional problems.

Index keyword: Childcare

Child Bereavement Trust, The

Aston House
High Street
West Wycombe
Bucks
HP14 3AG

Admin tel: 01494 446648
Admin fax: 01494 440057
Website: www.childbereavement.co.uk
E-mail: enquiries@childbereavement.co.uk

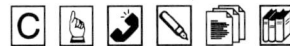

[icons]

Description: Offers training programmes for professionals and resources for bereaved families after the death of a child. Resources for families include leaflets, books and videos, but are not a counselling service.

Index keyword: Bereavement

Child Death Helpline

Great Ormond Street Hospital
for Children NHS Trust
London
WC1N 3JH

Helpline tel: 0800 282986
Admin tel: 020 7813 8550; 020 7813 8551
Admin fax: 020 7813 8516

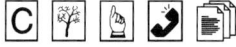

Description: This is a confidential helpline staffed almost entirely by bereaved parents, offering befriending and support to anyone affected by the death of a child.

Index keyword: Bereavement

Child Growth Foundation

2 Mayfield Avenue
Chiswick
London
W4 1PW

Helpline tel: 020 8995 0257
Admin tel: 020 8995 0257
Admin fax: 020 8995 9075

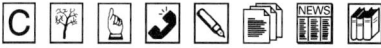

Description: Cares for children who grow too little or too much. Funds research, organises educational programmes and markets measuring equipment. Acts as an umbrella organisation for the Growth Hormone Insufficiency Group, Turner Syndrome, IUGR/Russell Silver, Bone Dysplasia, SOTOS and Premature Sexual Maturation support groups for patients and parents.

Index keyword: Growth Problems

Child Psychotherapy Trust, The

Star House
104–108 Grafton Road
London
NW5 4BD

Admin tel: 020 7284 1355
Admin fax: 020 7284 2755
E-mail: cpt@globalnet.co.uk

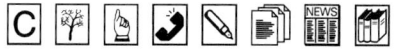

Description: The Child Psychotherapy Trust is a UK charity, established in 1987, dedicated to improving the lives of emotionally damaged children by increasing their access to child and adolescent psychotherapy services.

Index keyword: Psychotherapy

Childlessness Overcome Through Surrogacy

Loandho Cottage
Lairg
Sutherland
IV27 4EF

Helpline tel: 01549 402401
Admin tel: 01549 402401
Admin fax: 01549 402401

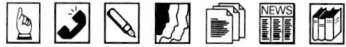

Description: Aims to help and support surrogates and couples and to give information to the public.

Index keyword: Pregnancy and Childbirth

Childline

2nd Floor,
Studd Street
London
N1 0QW

Helpline tel: 0800 1111
Admin tel: 020 7239 1000
Admin fax: 020 7239 1001
Website: www.childline.org.uk
Opening times: 24 hours

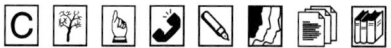

Description: ChildLine is the free, national helpline for children and young people in danger and distress. It provides a confidential phone counselling service for any child with any problem 24 hours a day, every day. It listens, comforts and protects. Trained counsellors provide support and advice and refer children in danger to appropriate helping agencies. ChildLine also brings to public attention issues affecting childrens' welfare and rights.

Index keyword: Children: General Information

Children's Chronic Arthritis Association

47 Battenhall Avenue
Worcester
WR5 2HN

Helpline tel: **01905 763556**
Admin tel: 01905 763556
Admin fax: 01905 763556
Website: www.ccaa.org.uk
Opening times: 8.30am–8.30pm

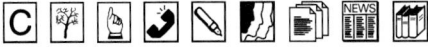

Description: Provides support and advice to children with arthritis and their families. Arranges and funds educational and recreational projects for them.

Index keyword: Arthritis/Rheumatic Disorders

Children's Head Injury Trust

c/o Neurosurgery
The Radcliffe Infirmary
Woodstock Road
Oxford
OX2 6HE

Helpline tel: **01865 224786**
Admin tel: 01865 224786
Admin fax: 01865 224786

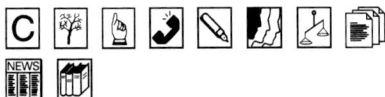

Description: The trust supports parents and head-injured children, and works to increase understanding in the community, create local family support groups, promote research and raise funds.

Index keyword: Head Injury

Children's Heart Federation

52 Kennington Oval
London
SE11 5SW

Helpline tel: **080 8085000**
Admin tel: 020 7820 8517
Admin fax: 020 7735 8718

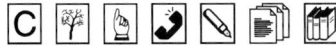

Description: Childrens' Heart Foundation is a charity providing a focus for groups which support children with heart disorder. It aims to encourage member groups to come together to exchange ideas and information, discuss common problems and work together to promote the interests of the children and families who make up the member groups.

Index keyword: Heart Problems

Children's Legal Centre Limited

University of Essex
Wivenhoe Park
Colchester
Essex
CO4 3SQ

Helpline tel: **01206 873820**
Admin tel: 01206 872466
Admin fax: 01206 874026
Website: www2.essex.ac.uk/clc
E-mail: clc@essex.ac.uk
Opening times: 10.00am–12.30pm, then 2.00pm–4.30pm

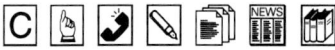

Description: Promotes and campaigns for the recognition of children and young people as individuals. Offers a free and confidential advice service, which covers all aspects of law and policy affecting young people and children. Open to adults and children.

Index keyword: Childcare

Children's Liver Disease Foundation

36 Great Charles Street
Birmingham
B3 3JY

Admin tel: 0121 212 3839
Admin fax: 0121 212 4300
Website: www.childliverdisease.org
E-mail: info@childliverdisease.org

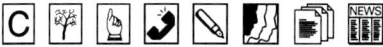

Description: Offers support, education and research by creating a greater awareness of paediatric liver disease; promoting research into its causes; developing early diagnosis, treatment and cures; providing new facilities and trained staff; ensuring emotional support for families of children with liver disease.

Index keyword: Liver Disease

Children's Trust, The

Tadworth Court
Tadworth
Surrey
KT20 5RU

Admin tel: 01737 357171
Admin fax: 01737 373848

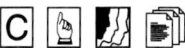

Description: Aims to provide care, treatment and education for children with

exceptional needs and profound disabilities and to give support to their families.

Index keyword: Disability: Children

Civil Service Benevolent Fund, The

Fund House
5 Anne Boleyn's Walk
Cheam, Sutton
Surrey
SM3 8DY

Helpline tel: **020 8240 2452**
Admin tel: 020 8240 2400
Admin fax: 020 8240 2401
Website: www.csbf.org.uk
E-mail: info@csbf.org.uk

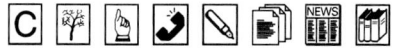

Description: The fund provides financial help and care to both serving and retire civil servants and staff of associated organisations and their dependants.

Index keyword: General Information

CLEANAIR (campaign for a smoke-free environment)

33 Stillness Road
London
SE23 1NG

Admin tel: 020 8690 4649
Website: www.azme.com/cleanair

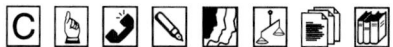

Description: Aims to create a smoke-free society for all to share and enjoy. Presents the latest scientific facts and expresses public opinion on smoking related issues.

Index keyword: Smoking

Climb

The Quadrangle
Crewe Hall
Weston Road
Crewe
Cheshire
CW1 6UR

Admin tel: 01270 250221
Admin fax: 01270 250244
Website: www.climb.org.uk

Description: Provides support and contact for parents of children suffering from inherited metabolic diseases and raises funds for research. Climb has information on 1300 rare inherited diseases and can put parents in touch with others. Also provides professional bodies with up-to-date information. Climb now provide support and an individual service to siblings and young adults.

Clearvision Project

Linden Lodge School
61 Princes Way
London
SW19 6JB

Admin tel: 020 8789 9575

Description: A nation-wide postal lending library of children's books with the brailled text interleaved on clear plastic sheets, so the books can be shared and enjoyed by blind and sighted children.

Index keywords: Blindness/Visual Handicap

Cleft Lip And Palate Association (CLAPA)

235–237 Finchley Road
London
NW3 6LS

Admin tel: 020 7431 0033
Admin fax: 020 7431 8881
Website: www.clapa.cwc.net
E-mail: clapa@cwcom.net

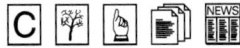

Description: Provides advice and support to the parents of children with cleft lip and/or palate, and subsequently to the children themselves.

Index keyword: Cleft Lip/Palate

CMT International UK

121 Lavernock Road
Penarth
South Wales
CF64 3QG

Admin tel: 029 2070 9537
Admin fax: 029 2070 9537

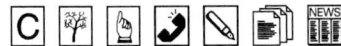

Description: This is a support group for people with Charcot-Marie-Tooth disease, also known as personal muscular atrophy and hereditary motor and sensory neuropathy. There are fundraising activities and events, and the group supports research into CMT. News letter also produced.

Index keyword: General Information

Coeliac Society, The

PO Box 220
High Wycombe
Bucks
HP11 2HY

Admin tel: 01494 437278
Admin fax: 01494 474349
Website: www.coeliac.co.uk
E-mail: admin@coeliac.co.uk

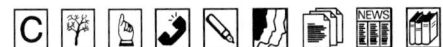

C

Description: This is a self-help group and charity, whose aim is to promote the welfare of those who have been medically diagnosed as having coeliac disease or dermatitis herpetiformis.

Index keyword: General Information

College of Osteopaths

13 Furzehill Road
Borehamwood
Hertfordshire
WD6 2DG

Admin tel: 020 8905 1937
Admin fax: 020 8953 7552

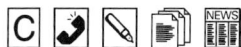

Description: The College of Osteopaths provides affordable holistic treatment, carried out by senior students under the close supervision of qualified osteopathic clinicians. Special rates for senior citizens, students and the unemployed.

Index keyword: Complementary Medicine

Colonic International Association

16 Drummond Ride
Tring
Herts
HP23 5DE

Admin tel: 01442 825632
Admin fax: 01442 827687
Website: www.colonic-association.com

Description: Informs the public about the benefits of colon hydrotherapy, protects them against untrained practitioners and sets training standards for colonic hydrotherapy. Publishes register of qualified colon hydrotherapists.

Index keywords: Complementary Medicine

Community Service Volunteers (CSV)

237 Pentonville Road
London
N1 9NJ

Helpline tel: **0800 374991**
Admin tel: 020 7278 6601
Admin fax: 020 7833 0149

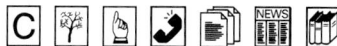

Description: CSV matches volunteers of all ages to full and part-time placements in health and social care settings.

Index keywords: Volunteers

Community Transport Association

Highbank
Halton Street
Hyde
Cheshire
SK14 2NY

Helpline tel: **0161 367 8780**
Admin tel: 0161 366 6685
Admin fax: 0161 366 6685
E-mail: cta.none@dial.pipex.com

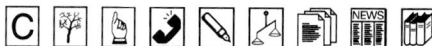

Description: Provides training, seminars and conferences on accessible transport provision.

Index keyword: Disability: General Information

Compassionate Friends, The

53 North Street
Bristol
BS3 1EN

Helpline tel: **0117 953 9639**
Admin tel: 0117 966 5202
Admin fax: 0117 966 5202

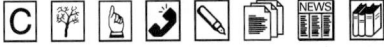

Description: This nationwide organisation of bereaved parents offers friendship and understanding to other bereaved parents after the death of a son or daughter from any cause. It provides personal and group support; support for bereaved siblings and grandparents; quarterly newsletter, postal library and range of leaflets. Befriending, rather than counselling.

Index keywords: Bereavement

Confederation of Healing Organisations

Red and White House
113 High Street
Berkhamsted
Hertfordshire
HP4 2DJ

Helpline tel: **01442 870660**
Admin tel: 01442 870660
Admin fax: 01442 870667

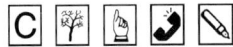

Description: Makes contact and distant healing available on the NHS and in Private medicine.

Index keywords: Complementary Medicine

Conquest (The Society for Art for Physically Handicapped People)

3 Beverley Close
East Ewell
Epsom
Surrey
KT12 3HB

Helpline tel: **020 8393 6102**
Admin tel: 020 8393 6102

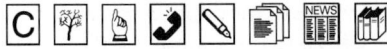

Description: The aims of Conquest are the relief and rehabilitation of physically disabled people by helping them to live full and more active lives and, wherever possible, assisting them to overcome their disability through participation in creative art activity. Art groups are set up, exhibitions organised, workshops held and talks given.

Index keywords: Disability: General Information

Consumers for Ethics in Research (CERES)

PO Box 1365
London
N16 0BW

E-mail: info@ceres.org.uk
Website: www.ceres.org.uk

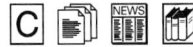

Description: More than half a million people a year in Britain take part in health research. CERES is concerned to publicise their views and to promote informed debate about research.

Index keyword: General Information

Contact a Family

170 Tottenhom Court Road
London
W1P 7HA

Admin tel: 020 7383 3555
Admin fax: 020 7383 0259
Website: www.cafamily.org.uk
E-mail: info@cafamily.org.uk

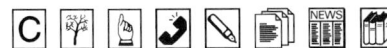

Description: Provides support, advice and information to families caring for children with any form of disability or special need. Helps parents' mutual support groups at national, regional and local levels.

Index keyword: Disability: Children

Continence Foundation (Incontinence Information Helpline)

307 Hatton Square
16 Baldwins Gardens
London
EC1N 7RJ

Admin tel: 020 7831 9831
Admin fax: 020 7404 6876
Website: www.continence-foundation.org.uk
E-mail: continence.foundation@dial.pipex.com

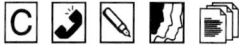

Ⓒ ☎ ✎ 👣 🗐

Description: The aim of the Continence Foundation Helpline is to encourage people whose lives are affected by incontinence to discuss their problem confidence with a trained.

Index keyword: Incontinence specialist nurse

Continuum

4A Hollybush Place
London
E2 9QX

Helpline: **020 7613 3909 (informal service)**
Admin tel: 020 7613 3909
Admin fax: 020 7613 3312
Website: www.continuum.org.uk
E-mail: continu@dircon.co.uk
Opening times: 11.00am–5.00pm

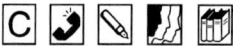

Ⓒ ☎ ✎ 👣 📑

Description: This is a pro-life organisation for long-term survivors of an HIV/AIDS diagnosis and those who want to be. It

produces a magazine promoting optimum health through nutrition and lifestyle changes, rather than orthodox medication. Also features alternative therapies, opinions and research, telephone advice and a monthly support group

Index keyword: AIDS and HIV

Convatec Limited

Harrington House
Milton Road
Ickenham
Uxbridge
UB10 8PU

Helpline tel: **0800 282254**
Admin tel: 01895 628300
Admin fax: 01895 628490

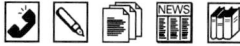

☎ ✎ 🗐 📰 📖

Description: Arranges roadshows, a series of spring and autumn events around the country, for ostomists, their families and healthcare professionals – a free day out with advice on up-to-date equipment and clothing, plus well-being advice on diet, style, etc.

Index keyword: General Information

Cope

Cope House
6 Tower Street
Leicester
LE1 6WS

Admin tel: 0116 254 9346
Admin fax: 0116 285 7481

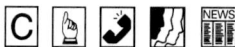

Ⓒ ☝ ☎ 👣 📰

Description: Aims to help children with cancer and to offer bereavement counseling to anyone who has lost a child through any cause

Index keyword: Cancer

Cornelia de Lange Syndrome Foundation

Tall Trees
106 lodge Lane
Grays
Essex
RM16 2UL

Admin tel: 01375 376439
Admin fax: 0702 5368998

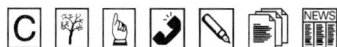

Description: The foundation is dedicated to ensuring early and accurate diagnosis of CdLS. Assists families, friends and professionals in making informed decisions and planning for the affected person's present and future. Promotes research, provides a support services for medical professionals and helps operate a network of interested professionals

Index keyword: Cornelia De Lange Syndrome

Coronary Artery Disease Research Association

121 Sydney Street
London
SW3 6NR

Helpline tel: 020 7349 8686
Admin tel: 020 7349 8686
Admin fax: 020 7349 9414

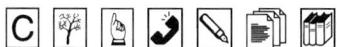

Description: Raises funds for research into the prevention of heart and arterial disease, with the aim of preventing premature death and disability.

Index keyword: Heart Problems

CORPAL

c/o John Cope-Faulkner
15 Burnt House Sidings
Pur
Whittlesey
Peterborough
PE7 2HS

Helpline tel: 01733 840073

Description: CORPAL is a support group for families who have a child with agenesis of the corpus callosum (ACC), including children with Aicardi's syndrome.

Index keyword: General Information

Cosmetic Surgery Network, The

PO Box 3410
London
N6 4EE

Helpline tel: 020 8209 0862
Admin tel: 020 8209 0862
Admin fax: 020 8983 3567
Website: www.cindyjackson.com

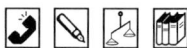

Description: Passes patient experiences and information on to prospective cosmetic surgery patients.

Index keyword: Cosmetic Surgery

Cot Death Society

Maple House
Unit 6/8
Padgate Business Centre
Green Lane
Warrington
Cheshire
WA1 4JN

Helpline: 0845 6010234
Admin tel: 01925 850086
Admin fax: 01925 851943
Website: www.cotdeathsociety.org.uk
E-mail: fundraising@cotdeath.society.org.uk
Opening times: 9.00am–5.00pm, Mon–Fri

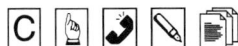

[icons]

Description: Provide a medical referral, infant respiration monitors for babies in the community at risk from cot death. The society also provides resuscitation video and guidelines on reducing the risk of cot death for parents and heart care professionals.

Cottage And Rural Enterprises Limited (CARE)

9 Weir Road
Kibworth
Leicester
LE8 OLQ

Admin tel: 0116 279 3225
Admin fax: 0116 279 6384
Website: www.care-ltd.co.uk
E-mail: carecentral@freeuk.com

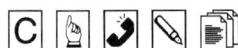

[icons]

Description: CARE is concerned with giving support, through the provision of residential accommodation and work facilities, to people who have a learning disability, and aims to offer each one the opportunity to live a full and purposeful life.

Index keyword: Mental Health/Illness

Council for Complementary and Alterative Medicine (CCAM)

206–208 Latimer Road
London
W10 6RE

Helpline tel: 020 8735 0632
Admin fax: 020 8968 3469
Opening times: 10am-5.30pm

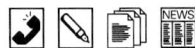

[icons]

Description: Aims to establish and maintain a forum for determining standards of education, training, ethics and discipline for practitioners of complementary therapy for the benefit of the public.

Index keyword: Complementary Medicine

Council for Disabled Children

8 Wakley Street
London
EC IV 7QE

Helpline tel: 020 7843 6058
Admin tel: 020 7843 6061
Admin fax: 020 7278 9512

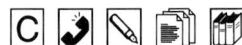

[icons]

Description: The Council for Disabled Children promotes collaborative work among organisations providing services and support for children and young people with disabilities and special educational needs.

Index keywords: Disability: Children

Council for Music in Hospitals

74 Queens Road
Hershom
Walton-on-Thames
Surrey
KT12 5LW

Admin tel: 01932 252809
Admin fax: 01932 252966

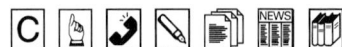

[icons]

Description: The Council provides around 4000 concerts in England, Wales and Northern Ireland, given by professional musicians.

Index keyword: Music

Council for the Advancement of Communication with Deaf People

Durham University Science Park
Block 4
Stockton Road
Durham
DH1 3UZ

Admin tel: 0191 383 1155
Admin fax: 0191 383 7914
Website: www.cacdp.demon.co.uk
E-mail: durham@cacdp.demon.co.uk

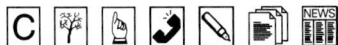

Description: CACDP is the national examining board for communication skills used between deaf and hearing people, including British sign language. lipspeaking, communicating with deafblind people and deaf awareness. Sells curricula for each of the examinations and produces sign language videos.

Index keyword: Hearing Problems/Deafness

Counsel and Care

Twyman House
16 Bonny Street
London
NW1 9PG

Helpline tel: 0845 3007585
Admin tel: 020 7485 1550
Admin fax: 020 7267 6877
E-mail: advice@counseland care.demon.co.uk
Opening times: 10.30 am–4.00pm, Weekdays

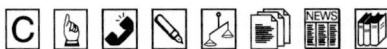

Description: Advises on a wide range of subjects, such as welfare benefits, accommodation, residential and nursing care. Maintains a database of home care agencies from which to advise individuals and are able to issue single payment grants for particular items.

Index keyword: Disability: Care Scheme/Holidays

Couple Counselling Scotland

40 North Castle Street
Edinburgh
EH2 3 BN

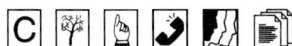

Helpline: 01382 640 340
Admin tel: 0131 225 5006
Admin fax: 0131 220 0639
Website: www.couplecounselling.org
Opening times: 2.00pm–4.00pm, Thurs

Description: Couple Counselling Scotland exists to promote, develop and co-ordinate counselling service for couples. Volunteers are professionally selected, trained, accredited and supervised throughout their time in CCS.

Index keyword: Couples Counselling

Craniofacial Support Group, The

44 Helmsdale Road
Leamington Spa
CV32 7DW

Helpline tel: 01926 334629
Admin tel: 01926 334629
Admin fax: 0870 133 9211

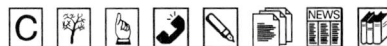

Description: Provides contact, information and mutual support to any family or individual where one of the 107 different syndromes or conditions presenting craniosynostosis is found.

Index keyword: Neurological

Cri du Chat Syndrome Support Group

7 Penny Lane
Barwell
Leicestershire
LE9 8HJ

Admin tel: 01455 841680

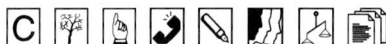

Description: Supports families and provides: information on the syndrome to carers and professionals; yearly get-togethers; research.

Index keyword: Cri Du Chat Syndrome

Criminal Injuries Compensation Authority

Tay House
300 Bath Street
Glasgow
G2 4LN

Helpline tel: **0141 331 2726**
Admin fax: 0141 331 2287

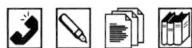

Description: The aim of the authority is to provide compensation for personal and fatal injuries sustained by innocent victims of crimes of violence.

Index keyword: Victims

Crisis Counselling for Alleged Shoplifters

PO Box 147
Stanmore
Middlesex
HA7 4PQ

Helpline tel: **020 8954 8987**
Admin tel: 020 7720 3685
Admin fax: 020 8385 3801

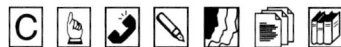

Description: Provides counselling and other general advice to persons accused of alleged shoplifting offences, for the purpose of giving moral support and general assistance; refers cases where expert assistance is required to a solicitor or social worker; has particular concern for children who may be accused; liaises with MPs, local authorities and other organisations to discuss aspects of policy and procedure.

Index keyword: Counselling

Crohn's in Childhood Research Association

Parkgate House
356 West Barnes Lane
Motspur Park
Surrey
KT3 6NB

Admin tel: 020 8949 6209
Admin fax: 020 8942 2044

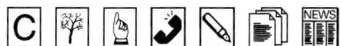

Description: Crohn's in Childhood raises funds for research into Crohn's disease, ulcerative colitis and related disorders (IBD). The Association offers help and understanding to suffers and their families. Information leaflets and regular newsletters are available for sufferers, parents, schools, health authorities and the medical profession.

Index keyword: Crohn's Disease

Crusaid

73 Collier Street
London
N1 9BE

Admin tel: 020 7833 3939
Admin fax: 020 7833 8644
Website: www.crusaid.org.uk
E-mail: office@crusaid.org.uk

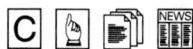

C 👆 📑 📰

Description: Crusaid helps men, women and children who are in dire financial needs as a result of HIV/AIDS to live a more dignified and fulfilling life. Funds AIDS-related projects, including education, housing, respite care, basic household bills, clothing etc. Each case is judged on its own merit.

Index keyword: AIDS and HIV

Cruse Bereavement Care (Northern Ireland)

Piney Ridge, Knockbracken Healthcare Park
Saintfield Road
Belfast
Northern Ireland
BT8 8BH

Admin tel: 02890 792419
Admin fax: 02890 792474

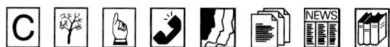

C 🌳 👆 📞 🦶 📑 📰 📖

Description: To support people who have been bereaved and to increase public awareness of the needs of bereaved people.

Index keyword: Death and Bereavement

Cruse Headquarters (Scotland)

33–35 Boswall Parkway
Edinburgh
EH5 2BR

Admin tel: 0131 551 1511
Admin fax: 0131 551 5234
E-mail: crusescothq@buzonline.co.uk

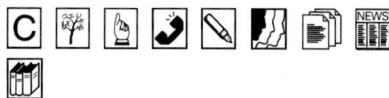

C 🌳 👆 📞 ✏ 🦶 📑 📰 📖

Description: Gives a nationwide service of the highest standard of counselling, information and social support to anyone who has been bereaved by death.

Index keyword: Death and Bereavement

('Serene') incorporating the Cry-sis Support Group

BM Cry-sis
London
WC1N 3XX

Helpline tel: 020 7404 5011
E-mail: serene@breathmail.net

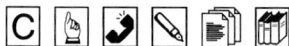

C 👆 📞 ✏ 📑 📖

Description: Offers self-help and support for families with excessively crying, sleepless and/or demanding young children. Support available by helpline and by post (sae please).

Index keyword: Children: General Information

Cult Information Centre

BCM Cults
London
WC1N 3XX

Helpline tel: 01689 833800

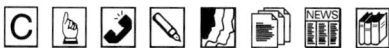

C 👆 📞 ✏ 🦶 📑 📰 📖

Description: Aims to increase awareness in society of the deceptive and psychologically coercive methods used by cults to recruit, indoctrinate and maintain membership. Gives talks, lectures and seminars to educational institutions, corporations, associations and the religious community on the dangers of cults. Assists individuals and families damaged by cults.

Index keyword: General Information

Cushing Care

Meadows
Woodplumpton Village
Preston
PR4 0LJ

Admin tel: 01772 690680
Admin fax: 01772 690680
E-mail: valhowarth@tinyworld.co.uk

Description: Aims to help people with Cushing's Disease/Syndrome, or their families, who need information or someone to talk to. Stamp addressed envelope for information, please.

Index keyword: Cushing Syndrome

Cypriot Advisory Service

26 Crowndale Road
London
NW1 1TT

Admin tel: 020 7387 6617
Admin fax: 020 7388 7971
E-mail: theatro.decsnis@virgin.net.

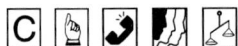

Description: Offers advice and support to Cypriot elderly people who have difficulty with the English language.

Index keyword: Ethnic Minorities

Cystic Fibrosis Trust

11 London Road
Bromley
Kent
BR1 1BY

Admin tel: 020 8464 7211
Admin fax: 020 8313 0472
Website: www.cftrust.org.uk
E-mail: enquiries@cftrust.org.uk
Opening times: 9.00am–5.00pm

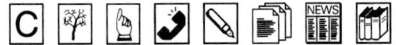

Description: The Cystic Fibrosis Trust medical and scientific research aimed at understanding, treating and curing Cystic Fibrosis. It also aims to ensure that people with Cystic Fibrosis receive the best possible care and support in all aspects of their lives.

Index keyword: Cystic Fibrosis

D

Dancing Eye Syndrome Support Group

78 Quantock Road
Worthing
West Sussex
BN13 2HQ

Admin tel: 01903 532383
Admin fax: 01903 532383
Website: www.mistral.co.uk
E-mail: rasr@mistral.co.uk

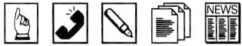

Description: Aims to provide support for families of children with dancing eye syndrome. The group organises a weekend break for families each year and an annual meeting for parents and professionals. The group also hopes to support a research programme in the future.

Index keyword: Eye Care

Dark Horse Venture

Kelton
Woodlands Road
Aigburth
Liverpool
L17 0AN

Admin tel: 0151 729 0092
Admin fax: 0151 729 0705

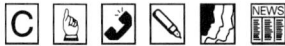

Description: The DHV is a national award scheme for retired and older people (55+). People are encouraged to take up activities such as sports, learning, volunteering, inter-generational work, and to achieve their personal best. Both active retired people and those with severe disabilities can join the scheme at little or no cost.

Index keyword: Elderly: General Information

David Lewis Organisation

Mill Lane
Warford
Near Alderley Edge
Cheshire
SK9 7UD

Admin tel: 01565 640000
Admin fax: 01565 640100

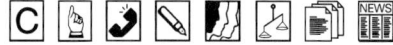

Description: Aims to maximise the quality of life for adults and children with epilepsy.

Index keyword: Epilepsy

Daycare Trust

Shoreditch Town Hall Annexe
380 Old Street
London
EC1V 9LT

Helpline tel: **020 7739 2866**
Admin tel: 020 7739 2866
Admin fax: 020 7739 5579

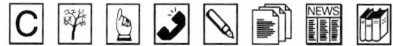

Description: Works to help parents find high quality, affordable childcare for their children, while the parents work or study; and to increase the provision of such childcare services, so that they become accessible to all who need them.

Index keyword: Childcare

Deaf Broadcasting Council

70 Blacketts Wood Drive
Chorleywood
Rickmansworth
Hertfordshire
WD3 5QQ

Admin tel: 01923 283127
Admin fax: 01923 283127

Website: deafbroadcastingcouncil.org.uk
E-mail: myers@waitrose.com

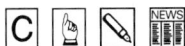

Description: A consumer organisation, to which the major organisations for hearing-impaired people are affiliated. Liaises with broadcasters to ensure that television and video are accessible to deaf, deafened and hard of hearing people and that access is of suitable quality. Activities cover the full range of televised broadcasting.

Index keyword: Hearing Problems/Deafness

Debendox Action Group

21 Corden Avenue
Mickleover
Derby
DE3 5AQ

Helpline tel: **01332 517896**
Admin tel: 01332 517896

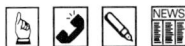

Description: Assists families in their endeavour to obtain compensation from the manufacturer of Debendox.

Index keyword: Drug Addiction/Side Effects

DEBRA

Debra House
13 Wellington Business Park
Dukes Ride
Crowthorne, Berkshire
RG45 6LS

Admin tel: 01344 771961
Admin fax: 01344 762661
Website: www.debra.org.uk
E-mail: debra.uk@btinternet.com

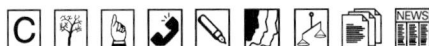

Description: Aims to promote the welfare of people with epidermolysis bullosa (EB) and to fund research into the condition. Funds specialist nursing and other healthcare staff to provide advice and assistance to people whose lives are affected by EB.

Index keyword: Skin Problems

Delta

PO Box 20
Haverhill
Suffolk
CB9 7BD

Helpline tel: **01440 783689**
Admin fax: 01440 783689
E-mail: deafeduc@aol.com

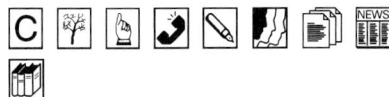

Description: A nationwide group of teachers and parents of deaf children which provides support, information and advice to guide parents in helping their deaf children to develop normal spoken language.

Index keyword: General Information

Dementia Services Development Centre

University of Stirling
Stirling
FK9 4LA

Admin tel: 01786 467740
Admin fax: 01786 466846
Website: www.stir.ac.uk/dsdc
E-mail: mt.calder@stir.ac.uk

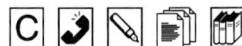

Description: The cutting edge of the centre's work is the development and consultancy service. The service has

THE HEALTH ADDRESS BOOK 2000–2001: A Directory of Health Support Groups

extensive experience of local, national and international services, plus knowledge gained from a wide body of literature and from conferences and seminars.

Index keyword: Mental Health/Illness

Department of Health (The Communicable Diseases Branch)

Room 655C
Skipton House
80 London Road,
London
SE1 6LH.

Helpline tel: 020 7972 5117
Admin tel: 020 7972 2000

Description: The branch handles policy on HIV and AIDS, on vaccination and immunisation and on other communicable diseases such as TB and hepatitis B. The establishment of this new branch continues the process by which HIV and AIDS are integrated into the mainstream of healthcare and health promotion.

Index keyword: AIDS and HIV

Depression Alliance

35 Westminister Bridge Road
London
SE1 7JB

Answer phone: 020 7633 9929
Admin tel: 020 7633 0557
Admin fax: 020 7633 0559
Website: www.depressionalliance.org
E-mail: hq@depressionalliance.org

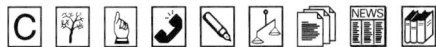

Description: Provision of information, and support to sufferers of depression and their carers, together with research into the causes of and treatments for depression and the dissemination of the results of such research.

Index keyword: Depression

Depressives Anonymous (Fellowship of)

Box FDA
Ormiston House
32–36 Peiham Street
Nottingham.
NG1 2EG

Information line: **01702 433838**
Admin fax: 01702 433843
Opening times: 9.00am–9.00pm

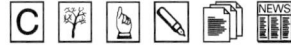

Description: Supports and encourages depressives and their families by informal contacts through its newsletter, penfriend scheme, local groups and public meetings. The aim is to shareexperiences and ease suffering.

Index keyword: Depression

DES Action UK

c/o Women's Health
52–54 Featherstone Street
London
EC1Y 8RT

Helpline tel: 020 7251 6580
Admin fax: 020 7608 0928
Website: www.womenslondonhealth.org.uk
E-mail: as website

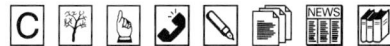

Description: Provides support and information to all those exposed to DES; also to the health profession.

Index keyword: DES Exposure

Dial UK

St Catherine's Hospital
Tickhill Road
Doncaster
DN4 8QN

Admin tel: 01302 310123
Admin fax: 01302 310404
Website: www.number.aol.com/dialuk
E-mail: dialuk@aol.com

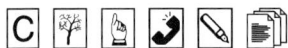

Description: This is a disability helpline.

Index keyword: Disability: General Information

DIEL (advisory committee on telecommunications for Disabled and Elderly people)

50 Ludgate Hill
London
EC4M 7JJ

Helpline tel: **020 7634 8770**
Admin tel: 020 7634 8770
Admin fax: 020 7634 8845

Description: DIEL promotes the needs of doubled and elderly telephone-users and provides an independent bridge between them and the telecommunications industry.

Index keyword: Disability: Equipment

Disabilities Trust (Formerly the Disabled Housing Trust)

1st Floor
32 Market Place
Burgess Hill
West Sussex
RH15 9NP

Admin tel: 01444 239123
Admin fax: 01444 244978
Website: www.disabilities-trust.org.uk
E-mail: info@disabilities-trust.org.uk

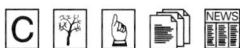

Description: The Disabilities Trust provides residential, respite and day facilities for those with severe physical disabilities, acquired brain injury or autism.

Index keyword: Disability: General Information

Disability Action

69 Church Road
Castleraegh
Belfast
BT6 9SA

Helpline tel: **02890 791900**
Admin tel: 02890 791900
Admin fax: 02890 791950
Text phone: 02890 645779
Website: www.disabilityaction.org
E-mail: hq@disabilityaction.org
Opening times: Mon-Fri 9am-5pm

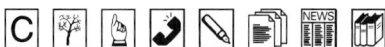

Description: Provides a means of consultation and joint action for organisations and individuals working for the well-being of people with disabilities. Provides information, training, support services, advice on access to the environment and transport services.

Index keyword: Disability: General Information

Disability Alliance

Universal House
88–94 Wentworth Street
London
E1 7SA

Helpline tel: **020 7247 8763 (Rights Advice Line)**
Admin tel: 020 7247 8776 (Ring this number for info on publications)

Admin fax: 020 7247 8765
Website: under construction

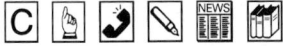

[C] [icons]

Description: Our aim is to break the link between poverty and disability. To do this we provide information for disabled people, about their entitlements through publications such as the *Disability Rights Handbook* and *The Rights Advice Line*.

Index keyword: Disability: General Information

Disability Benefits Unit

Warbreck House
Warbreck Hill
Blackpool
FY5 3AW

Helpline tel: 0845 7123456
Benefit Enquiry tel: 0800 882200
Admin fax: 01253 331266
E-mail: dbu-customerservice@ms24.dss.gov.uk

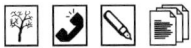

[icons]

Description: Administers attendance and disability living allowances, ensuring that payment is made at the correct rate to the right person at the right time.

Index keyword: Disability: General Information

Disability Equipment Register

4 Chatterton Road
Yate
Bristol
BS37 4BJ

Admin tel: 01454 318818
Admin fax: 01454 883870
Website: www.disabreg.dial.pipex.com
E-mail: disabreg@dial.pipex.com

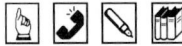

[icons]

Description: The register is a service for disabled people and their families, enabling them to buy, sell or exchange used specialist equipment without having to pay advertising fees.

Index keyword: Disability: Equipment

Disability Information Trust

Mary Marlborough Centre,
Nuffield Orthopedics Centre
Headington
Oxford
OX3 7LD

Admin tel: 01865 227592
Admin fax: 01865 227596
Website: www.home.btconnect.com/ditrust/home.htm
E-mail: www.ditrust@btconnect.com

[C] [icon]

Description: The trust assesses and tests a wide range of disability equipment and publishes independent in-depth information on the items evaluated in its series of books

Index keyword: Disability: Equipment

Disability Sport England

13–27 Brunswick Place
London
N1 6DX

Helpline: 020 7490 4919
Admin fax: 020 7490 4914
Website: www.britsport.com
E-mail: infor@dse.org.com
Opening times: 10.00am–4.00pm

Disability Wales (Anableddcymru)

Llys Ifor
Crescent Road
Caerphilly
CF83 1XL

Admin tel: 02920 887325
Admin fax: 02920 888702
E-mail: info@dwac.demon.co.uk

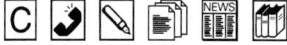

C 🎧 📝 🗐 📰 📊

Description: Works to promote the rights, recognition and support of all disabled people in Wales.

Index keyword: Disability: General Information

Disabled Christians Fellowship, The

213 Wick Road
Brislington
Bristol
BS4 4HP

Helpline tel: **0117 983 0388**
Admin tel: 0117 983 0388
Admin fax: 0117 914 8910
E-mail: dcf@dcfbristol.freeserve.co.uk

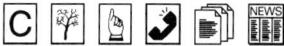

C 🌳 ✋ 🎧 🗐 📰

Description: The aim of the Disabled Christians Fellowship is to bring ability into disability within a Christian environment

Index keyword: Disability: General Information

Disabled Drivers Association, The

National Headquarters
Ashwellthorpe
Norwich
NR 16 1EX

Admin tel: 01508 489449
Admin fax: 01508 488173
Website: www.justmobility.co.uk/dda
E-mail: ddahq@aol.com

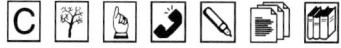

C 🌳 ✋ 🎧 📝 🗐 📊

Description: DDA seeks to maintain a full information service. Assists in finding solutions to members' problems. Campaigns through liaison with government and local bodies to advance the cause of disabled people.

Concessions with many ferry companies. Advice on local activities to members.

Index keyword: Disability: General Information

Disabled Drivers Motor Club

Cottingham Way
Thrapston
Northamptonshire
NN14 4PL

Helpline tel: **01832 734724**
Admin tel: 01832 734724
Admin fax: 01832 733816
Website: www.ukonline.co.uk.ddmc
E-mail: ddmc@ukonline.co.uk

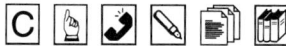

C ✋ 🎧 📝 🗐 📊

Description: The DDMC is a registered charity actively campaigning for greater mobility and better access for all disabled people on the move.

Index keyword: Disability: Equipment

Disabled Motorists Federation

41 Weston Drive
Cheslyn Hay
Walsall
West Midlands
WS6 7NQ

Helpline tel: **0191 4163172**

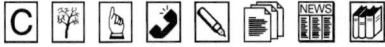

Description: Aims to better the quality of life and mobility of disabled drivers.

Index keyword: Disability: General Information

Disabled Parents Network

PO Box 5876
Towcester
NN12 7ZN

Helpline tel: **0870 241 0450**
Admin tel: 020 8992 8637
Admin fax: 020 8992 5929

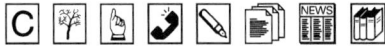

Description: Disabled Parents Network is a National Childbirth Trust network of disabled parents. It supports them in pregnancy, childbirth and parenthood.

Index keyword: Pregnancy and Childbirth

Disabled Photographers Society

General Secretary
26 St Leonards Avenue
Chineham
Basingstoke
Hampshire
RG24 8RD

Admin tel: 01256 351990
Admin fax: 01256 351990

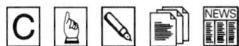

Description: Encourages disabled and handicapped people to take an active interest in photography as a therapeutic and creative pursuit.

Index keyword: Disability: General Information

Disablement Income Group Scotland

5 Quayside Street
Edinburgh
EH6 6EJ

Helpline tel: **0131 555 2811**
Admin fax: 0131 554 7076

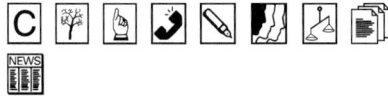

Description: A national charity providing free information and advice on welfare benefits to disabled people and carers in Scotland. Membership £5 per year (optional).

Index keyword: Disability: General Information

Disablement Income Group, The

PO Box 5743
Finchingfield
CM7 4PW

Helpline tel: **01371 811621**
Admin fax: 01371 811633

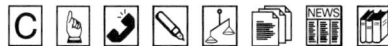

Description: The Disablement Income Group is a national campaigning charity promoting the financial welfare of disabled people through a programme of advice, advocacy, fieldwork, information, publications, research and training.

Index keyword: Disability: General Information

Disability Law Service

39–45 Cavell Street
London
E1 2BP

Helpline tel: **020 7791 3131**
Admin tel: 020 7791 9800

Admin fax: 020 7791 9802
Minicom: 020 7791 9801

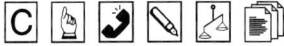

[C] [☞] [☎] [✎] [♿] [🗐]

Description: Gives free legal advice and representation to disabled people and their families and/or carers throughout Britain. Advice on benefits, community care, discrimination, education, employment, housing, wills and trusts, and numerous other matters which affect the lives of disabled people.

Index keyword: Disability: General Information
Mrs Anderson

DISCERN

Chadburn House
Weighbridge Road
Littleworth
Mansfield
Notts
NG18 1AH

Helpline tel: 01623 623732
Admin fax: 01623 623732

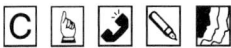

[C] [☞] [☎] [✎] [🏃]

Description: DISCERN offers a confidential counselling service to people with physical desabilities or learning difficulties who wish to explore issues around their sexuality and personal relationships. DISCERN also provides a staff training service and a consultancy service.

Index keyword: Disability: General Information

Disfigurement Guidance Centre

PO Box 7
Cupar
Fife
KY15 4PF
Admin tel: 01337 870281
Admin fax: 01337 870310

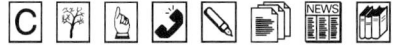

[C] [🌳] [☞] [☎] [✎] [🗐] [NEWS] [📖]

Description: Over the last 30 years the DGC has targeted different areas to meet major needs in the field of disfigurement. For example, the DGC's last project, Laserfair, brought the new generation of skin lasers to the UK and established six, new NHS laser clinics. Literature also available to Doctors/public on request. A small fee

Index keyword: Disfigurement

Donor Conception Network

PO Box 265
Sheffield
S3 7YX

Admin tel: 020 8245 4369
Website: www.dinetwork.org.uk
E-mail:
101603.2644@compuserve.com/dinetwork

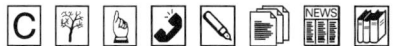

[C] [🌳] [☞] [☎] [✎] [🗐] [NEWS] [📖]

Description: Aims to provide support to existing parents, to their children, and to those contemplating or undergoing DI treatment. Holds national and local meetings.

Index keyword: Infertility

Douglas Bader Centre

The Douglas Bader Centre
Roehampton Lane
London
SW15 5DZ

Admin tel: 020 8788 1551
Admin fax: 020 8789 5622

Description: The centre has a sports hall
and gym where the machines are
designed to be wheel-chair friendly (no
need to transfer). The centre is open to
both able-bodied and disabled people.
Special training programmes can be
worked out by the fully qualified staff.
The centre also caters for people wishing
to do cardio-vascular programmes to
lose weight and keep fit, whatever their
age.

Index keyword: Disability: Sport/
Exercise

Down's Syndrome Association

155 Mitcham Road
London
SW17 9PG

Admin tel: 020 8682 4001
Admin fax: 020 8682 4012
Website: www.downs-syndrome.org.uk
E-mail: info@downs-syndrome.org.uk

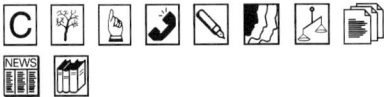

Description: Offers advice, support and
counselling to people with Down's
Syndrome, their parents, carers,
interested professionals and others.
Funds research into various aspects of
living with Down's Syndrome.

Index keyword: Down's Syndrome

Dr Edward Bach Centre

Mount Vemon
Baker's Lane
Sotwell.
Oxen
OX10 0PZ
01491 834 678
9:30am–4:30pm

Helpline tel: **01491 834678**
Admin fax: 01491 825022
Website: www.bachcentre.com
E-mail: mail@bachcentre.com
Opening hours: 9.30am–4.30pm

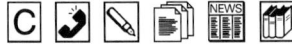

Description: The Bach Flower Remedies are
38 remedies used against the negative
emotional states that can be the cause of
illness. The Bach Centre was Dr Bach's
home, where the remedies are will
prepared according to his instructions. The
Centre provides education and information
and a list of registered practitioners.

Index keyword: Complementary Medicine

Dr Jan de Winter Cancer Prevention Foundation

6 New Road
Brighton
East Sussex
BN1 1UF

Helpline tel: **01273 727213**
Admin tel: 01273 727213
Admin fax: 01273 748915
Website: www.brightonclinic.freeserve.co.uk
E-mail:
drjandewinter@brightonclinic.freeserve.co.uk

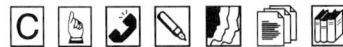

Description: Works for prevention of cancer
and heart disease through advancement of
public education in health. Early detection
facilities for cancer, heart disease, high
blood pressure, stroke, diabetes and
osteoporosis. Counselling for stress
avoidance. Advice on relief of menopausal

symptoms, including advisability of HRT and non-hormonal means.

Index keyword: Cancer

Dreamflight

3 Saxeway
Chartridge Lane
Chartridge
Bucks
HP5 2SH

Helpline tel: **01494 792991**
Admin tel: 01494 792991
Admin fax: 01494 775211
Website: www.dreamflight.org
E-mail: dreamflight@compuserve.com

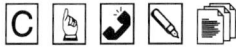

Description: Takes 192 seriously ill or disabled children on a week-long holiday of a lifetime to Orlando, with the aim of bringing some fun and joy into the lives of children who have suffered a lot through illness and treatment.

Index keyword: Disability: Care Scheme/Holidays

Drinkline

1st Floor
Cavern Court
8 Matthew Street
Liverpool
L2 6RE

Helpline tel: **0800 917 8282**
Admin fax: 0151 227 4019

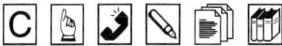

Description: Drinkline's objectives are to educate callers about alcohol; advise callers on appropriate services and other forms of help; help callers who are worried about their own drinking; support the family and friends of people who are drinking.

Index keyword: Alcohol Problems

Drugcare

29 Upper Lattimore Road
St Albans
Hertfordshire
AL1 3UA

Helpline tel: **01727 834539**
Admin tel: 01727 861084
Admin fax: 01727 834667
Opening hours: 10.00am–1.00pm and 2.00pm–4.00pm, Mon–Fri and outside these hours by appointment.

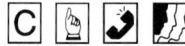

Description: Aims to give practical help, support and advice to any person who sees drugs as a problem, either directly or as family member or friend. Other activities: daily drop-in, needle exchange, relaxation sessions, complementary therapies.

Index keyword: Drug Addiction/Side Effects

Dystonia Society, The

46–47 Britton Street
London
EC1M 5UJ

Helpline tel: **020 7490 5671**
Admin tel: 020 7490 5671
Admin fax: 020 7490 5672

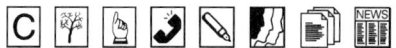

Description: Supports people who have any form of the neurological movement disorder known as dystonia, and their families, through the promotion of awareness, research and welfare.

Index Keyword: Dystonia

E

Eating Disorders Association

1st Floor
Wensum House
103 Prince of Wales Road
Norwich
Norfolk
NR1 1DW

Helpline tel: 01603 621414
Admin tel: 01603 619090
Admin fax: 01603 664915

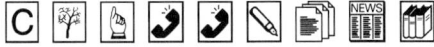

[C] [icons]

Description: Provides support and information to people with eating disorders, their families and carers. Local groups, local help, membership scheme and information are available.

Index keyword: Eating Disorders

Edward's Trust

Edward House
St Marys Row, off Whittall Street
Birmingham
B4 6NY

Helpline tel: 0121 454 1705

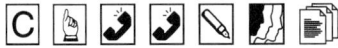

[C] [icons]

Description: The Trust was set up to promote the relief of children with cancer and of families who have suffered the death of a child from conception onwards; to increase awareness in the family of complementary approaches to childhood cancers; to support research into childhood cancers and disseminate the useful results.

Index keyword: Cancer

Ehlers-Danlos Syndrome Support Group

PO Box 335
Farnham
Surrey
GU10 1XJ

Admin tel: 01252 690940
Admin fax: 01252 404573

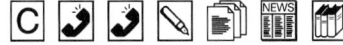

[C] [icons]

Description: Aims to help, encourage and inform people with EDS and their family members. Links members with one another for mutual support and the rechange of ideas. Maintains a list of specialists who have a particular interest art and experience of, the condition.

Index keyword: Ehlers-Danlos Syndrome

Eileen Trust, The

Alliance House
12 Caxton Street
London
SW1H 0QS

Admin tel: 020 7799 3184
Admin fax: 020 7233 0839

[C] [icon]

Description: Offers support to people other than those with haemophilia) who were infected with HIV by contaminated blood or tissue transfer in the UK.

Index keyword: AIDS and HIV

Elderly Accommodation Council

3rd Floor
89 Albert Embankment
London
SE1 7TP

Admin tel: 020 7820 1343

Admin fax: 020 7820 3970
E-mail: enquiries@e-a-c.demon.co.uk

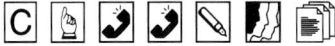

C ☞ ✆ ✆ ✎ ☘ 🗐

Description: Elderly Accommodation Counsel is a registered charity which maintains a nationwide database of all forms of accommodation for older people, sheltered housing for sale and rent, residential care homes, nursing homes and close care schemes. Staff also give guidance, advice and detailed information to help enquirers choose and find the accommodation most suited to their needs.

Index keyword: Elderly: Accommodation/Housing

Electronic Aids for the Blind

Suite 4b, 71–75 High Street
Chislehurst
Kent
BR7 5AG

Admin tel: 020 8295 3636
Admin fax: 020 8295 3737

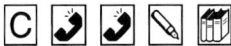

C ✆ ✆ ✎ 📖

Description: This national charity works to enhance the independence and levels of achievement for blind and partially-sighted people, through the provision of specialist or suitably adapted electronic equipment. Undertakes fund-raising for such equipment on behalf of individuals where no statutory or personal resources exist.

Index keyword: Blindness/Visual Handicap

Elizabeth Finn Trust, The

1 Derry Street
London
W8 5HY

Helpline tel:
Admin tel: 020 7396 6700
Admin fax: 020 7396 6739

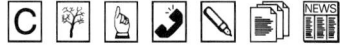

C 🌳 ☞ ✆ ✎ 🗐 📰

Description: Nursing and residential homes are located in Exeter, Virginia Water, Woodbridge, Eastbourne, Tunbridge Wells, London, Droitwich, Wallingford, Harrogate. Grants and one-off gifts are made to people from professional backgrounds who have fallen on hard times.

Index keyword: Elderly: Accommodation/Housing

Elizabeth House Association

209 Ladbroke Grove
London
W10 6HQ

Helpline tel: 020 7243 0372
Admin tel: 020 7243 0372

C ☞ ✆

Description: The Elizabeth House Association offers residential care for former drug-users who wish to live a drug-free life. Offers a full range of services, from detoxification to independent living.

Index keyword: Drug Addiction/Side Effects

Enable

6th Floor
7 Buchanan Street
Glasgow
G1 3HL

Helpline tel: 0141 226 4541
Admin fax: 0141 204 4398
E-mail: enable@enable.org.uk

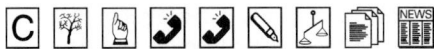

Description: ENABLE is the largest voluntary organisation in Scotland which represents the interests of people with learning disabilities. Formed by parents in 1954, it has over 70 branches across Scotland and a membership of around 6000. Membership and campaigning services include information and legal advice and support for families. ENABLE Services provides holidays, jobs, training, day services and respite care, while ENABLE Homes has 12 family-sized homes for people with profound and complex needs.

Index keyword: Disability: General Information

Encephalitis Support Group

44a Market
Malton
N. Yorks
YO17 7LW

Helpline tel: **01653 699599**
Admin tel: 01653 699599
Admin fax: 01653 699599

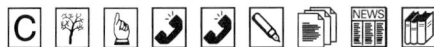

Description: The Group supports sufferers of encephalitis and their families in dealing with the long-term after effects. It works to raise awareness of the condition and to raise funds for research.

Index keyword: Encephailitis

Epilepsy and the Young Adult (EYA)

13 Crondace Road
London
SW6 4BB

Admin tel: 020 7736 0123
Admin fax: 020 7736 4118

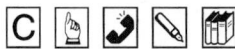

Description: EYA's aim is the continued production of *Epilepsy and the Young Adult*, a booklet which provides comprehensive information and advice for young people living with epilepsy. *See* Epilepsy Bereaved.

Index keyword: Epilepsy

Epilepsy Association of Scotland

48 Govan Road
Glasgow
G51 1JL

Helpline tel: **0141 427 4911**
Admin tel: 0141 427 4911
Admin fax: 0141 427 7414/419 1709
Website: www.epilepsyscotland.org.uk
E-mail: support@epilepsyscotland.org.uk

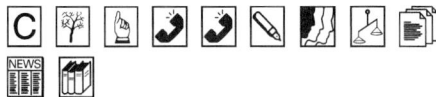

Description: Promotes the welfare and well-being of people with epilepsy. Activities and services include: information, advice, support and counselling services; social work, field and community projects; promoting public education about epilepsy; training a wide range of professional groups in understanding and managing epilepsy.

Index keyword: Epilepsy

Epilepsy Bereaved

PO Box 112
Wantage P.O.
OX12 8XT

Helpline: **01235 772852**
Admin tel: 01235 772850
Website: dspace.dial.pipex.com/epilepsybereaved
E-mail: epilepsybereaved@dial.pipex.com

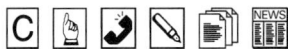

Description: The charity is a self-help group for mutual support and unformation. It seeks to aid reserach and raise awareness of sudden, unexpected death in epilepsy.

Index keyword: Epilepsy

Epoch (End Physical Punishment of Children)

77 Holloway Road
London
N7 8JZ

Admin tel: 020 7700 0627
Admin fax: 020 7700 1105
E-mail: epoch-worldwide@mcrl.poptel.org.uk

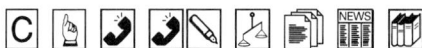

Description: EPOCH was launched in 1989 as a national campaign to end physical punishment of children. The campaign is supported by over 60 organisations in the children's field. It hopes to achieve its aim through education, research and legal reform.

Index keyword: Childcare

Erb's Palsy Group

2 Willoughby Close
Coventry
Warwickshire
CV3 2GJ

Helpline tel: **024 7645 2321**
Admin tel: 01442 212422
Admin fax: 0247 645 3366

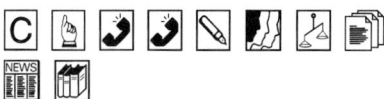

Description: Helps and supports parents by putting them in contact with one

another. Produces a newsletter, assists in obtaining medical information, advises on benefits and aids for children and has annual social get-togethers for families. Also has an annual information day for professionals.

Index keyword: Childcare

Evelina Children's Heart Organisation (ECHO)

3 Lincolnshire Terrace
Lane End
Dartford
Kent
DA2 7JP

Helpline tel: **01424 813785**
Admin tel: 01424 813785

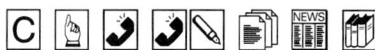

Description: Aims to put parents in touch with one another for mutual help and support; to constitute a link and a means of communication between parents and staff; to raise funds to buy equipment and resources for the comfort of both children and relatives to organise events for the benefit of children and hospital.

Index keyword: Heart Problems

Ex-Services Mental Welfare Society

Head Office
Tyrwhitt House
Oaklawn House
Leatherhead
Surrey
KT22 0BX

Helpline tel: **01372 841600**
Admin fax: 01372 841601
Website: www.combatstress.com
E-mail: ESMWS@aol.com

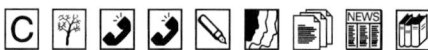

Description: The society specialises in the care of men and women of all ranks discharged from the armed services and merchant navy who suffer from injury to the mind. There is a regional network of welfare officers throughout the country.

Index keyword: Mental Health/Illness

EXCEL 2000

1a North Street
Sheringham
Norfolk
NR26 8LW

Admin tel: 01263 825670

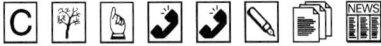

Description: Offers exercise with ease and enjoyment, relaxation and training in body awareness. Aims to provide services and support, information and advice, for all people with special needs and their carers, of all ages and cultures.

Index keyword: Disability: Sport/Excercise

Extend Exercise Training Limited

22 Maltings Drive
Wheathampstead
Hertfordshire
AL4 8QJ

Helpline tel: **01582 832760**
Admin tel: 01582 832760
Admin fax: 01582 832760
Website: www.extend.org.uk
E-mail: admin@extend.org.uk

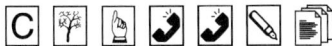

Description: Provides recreational movement to music for the over-60s and for less able people of any age. There is Extend exercise classes in various areas of the UK.

Index keyword: Elderly: General Information

FAB-UK

4 Pateley Road
Woodthorpe
Nottingham
NG3 5QF

Helpline tel: **0115 926 9634**
Opening times: Daily 10am-10pm

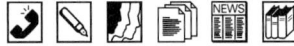

Description: FAB-UK is a contact group for families of children with Fanconi's Anaemia and professionals with an interest in the condition. The group provides support and information among families, information updates on the condition and undertakes fundraising to assist research into bone marrow transplants.

Index keyword: Children: General Information

Fabry Disease Research Fund and Support Group

10 Broadmeadow Road
Wyke Regis
Weymouth
DT4 9BS

Helpline tel: **01305 774443**
Admin tel: 01305 774443
Admin fax: 01305 774443
E-mail: fabry@wdi.co.uk

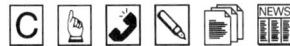

Description: Aims to promote awareness of Fabry disease and to raise money for search.

Index keyword: Fabry's Disease

Faculty of Homoeopathy

15 Clerkenwell Close
London
EC1R 0AA

Admin tel: 020 7566 7800
Admin fax: 020 7566 7815
E-mail: info@trusthomeopathy.org

Description: This is a professional body for registered healthcare practitioners who have completed additional training a homoeopathy. The faculty is responsible for maintaining standards of training and education in homoeopathy for healthcare professionals.

Index keyword: Complementary Medicine

Faithfully Yours

15 St Oswalds Crescent
Billingham
TS23 2RW

Description: Offers comfort, help and advice to people who have been bereaved of their pets. Free advice is given to any age group after loss of any type of animal.

Index keyword: Bereavement

Families Anonymous

37 The Doddington-Rollo Community Association
Charlotte Despard Avenue
Battersea
London
SW11 5JE

Helpline tel: 020 7498 4680
Admin tel: 020 7498 4680
Admin fax: 020 7498 1990
Website: www.famanon.org.uk

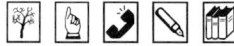

Description: Gives support to families and friends of people who use and abuse drugs. Provides literature and self help groups throughout UK.

Index keyword: Drug Addiction/Side Effects

Families Need Fathers

134 Curtain Road
London
EC2A 3AR

Helpline tel: 020 7613 5060
Admin tel: 020 7613 5060
Website: www.fnf.org.uk

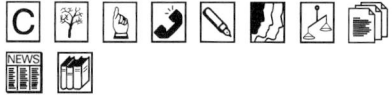

Description: Keeping children in contact with both parents, following divorce or separation.

Index keyword: Divorce/Separation

Family Action Information and Resource (FAIR)

BCM Box 3535
PO Box 12
London
WC1N 3XX

Admin tel: 01642 898412
Admin fax: 01642 643707

Description: Provides counselling and information for families adversely affected by their children's involvement in extremist religious cults. Counselling (with consent) for members and ex-members of such groups.

Index keyword: Family Support and Welfare

Family Care

21 Castle Street
Edinburgh
EH2 3DN

Helpline tel: **0131 225 6441**
Admin tel: 0131 225 6478
Admin fax: 0131 225 6478
E-mail: family.care@virgin.net

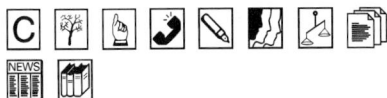

Description: Family Care helps vulnerable
children and families, especially through:
Birth Link, an adoption contact register
and other services for anyone involved in
an adoption (birth parents and relatives,
adopted people, adoptive families);
counselling for children and for parents;
befriending and other practical help.

Index keyword: Adoption and Fostering

Family Fund Trust, The

PO Box 50
York
YO1 2ZX

Helpline tel: **01904 621115**
Admin tel: 01904 621115
Admin fax: 01904 652625
Website: www.familyfundtrust.org.uk
E-mail: same as website

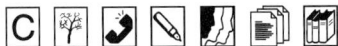

Description: The purpose of the trust is to
ease the stress on families who care for
very severely disabled children under 16,
by providing grants and information
related to the care of the child. Grants
include laundry equipment, holidays,
outings, driving lessons, bedding and
clothing.

Index keyword: Disability: Children

Family Heart Association

7 North Road
Maidenhead
Berks
SL6 1PE

Admin tel: 01628 628638
Admin fax: 01628 628698

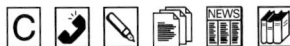

Description: Provides information and
help for people with inherited high
cholesterol levels or who are prone to
premature angina or heart attack for other
reasons.

Index keyword: Heart Problems

Family Planning Association

2–12 Pentonville Road
London
N1 9FP

Helpline tel: **020 7837 4044**
Admin tel: 020 7837 5432
Admin fax: 020 7837 3042

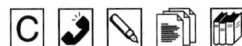

Description: Promotes sexual and
reproductive health and rights.

Index keyword: General Information

Family Planning Association Scotland

Unit 10
Firhill Business Centre
74 Firhill Road
Glasgow
G20 7BA

Helpline tel: **0141 576 5088**
Admin tel: 0141 576 5088
Admin fax: 0141 576 5006

Website: www.fpa.org.uk
Opening hours: 9.00am–5.00pm,
Mon–Thurs; 9.00am–4.30pm, Fri.

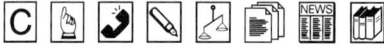

C 👆 📞 ✏️ 📐 📑 📰 📖

Description: FPA works to advance the sexual health and reproductive rights and choices of all people throughout the UK.

Index keyword: Family Planning

Family Planning Association Wales

Ground Floor
Riverside House
31 Cathederal Road
Cardiff
CF11 9HB

Admin tel: 02920 644034
Admin fax: 02920 644306
E-mail: fpa@cymru@compuserve.com

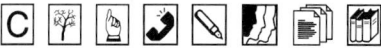

C 🌳 👆 📞 ✏️ 🦶 📑 📖

Description: Aims to advance the sexual health and reproductive rights and choices of all people throughout the UK. FPA Cymru provides training for professionals, sex education, community education, consultancy, helpline for clinic information and around relationships, sexuality, contraception, etc.

Index keyword: Family Planning

Family Policy Studies Centre

9 Tavistock Place
London
WC1H 9SN

Admin tel: 020 7388 5900
Admin fax: 020 7388 5600

C 📰 📖

Description: The centre is an independent body, whose primary concern is social policy and the family. It is a centre of research and information, which publishes reports and a bulletin and maintains a small library.

Index keyword: General Information

Family Service Units

207 Old Marylebone Road
London
NW1 5QP

Admin tel: 020 7402 5175
Admin fax: 020 7724 1829
E-mail: centraloffice@fsu.org.uk

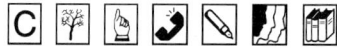

C 🌳 👆 📞 ✏️ 🦶 📖

Description: This national voluntary social work agency supports families and children living in communities in the greatest need, so they can draw on their own strengths and take control of their lives. FSU strives to address wider injustices and influences that prevent families from achieving their potential.

Index keyword: Family Support and Welfare

Family Welfare Association

501–5 Kingsland Road
London
E8 4AU

Admin tel: 020 7254 6251
Admin fax: 020 7249 5443

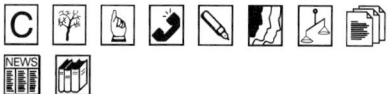

C 🌳 👆 📞 ✏️ 🦶 📐 📑 📰 📖

Description: FWA provides practical, financial and social care to families: grant-giving, community mental health services and family support services.

Index keyword: Family Support and Welfare

Federation of Multiple Sclerosis Therapy Centres

MS Service Centre
Bradbury House
155 Barkers Lane
Bedford
MK41 9RX

Admin tel: 01234 325781
Admin fax: 01234 365242
Website: www.ms-selfhelp.org
E-mail: info@ms-selfhelp.org

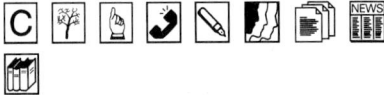

Description: Provides information, support and training to the MS therapy centres within the federation. These provide professional therapy to MS sufferers, plus information, including a diet booklet, and support.

Index keyword: Multiple Sclerosis

Fertility UK

Clitherow House
1 Blythe Mews
Blythe Road
London
W14 ONW

Helpline tel: **020 7371 1341**
Admin tel: 020 7371 1341
Admin fax: 020 7371 4921
Website: www.fertilityuk.org
E-mail: admin@fertilityuk.org

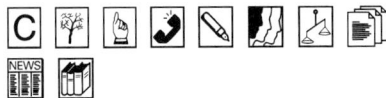

Description: Provides an educational service giving practical instruction in fertility awareness and the sympto-thermal method of natural family planing (NFP). Fertility awareness education can be used to achieve pregnancy and is particularly beneficial for sub-fertile couples. NFP is a highly effective means of avoiding pregnancy. The organisation also provides speakers for NHS family planning courses and university accredited training for health professionals.

Index keyword: Family Planning and Infertility

First Steps to Freedom

7 Avon Court
School Lane
Kenilworth
Warwickshire
CV8 2GX

Helpline tel: **01926 851608**
Admin tel: 01926 851608
Admin fax: 01926 864473
Website: www.firststeps.demon.co.uk
E-mail: firststepstofreedom@compuserve.com
Opening hours: 10.00am–10.00pm, daily

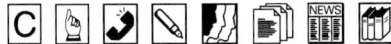

Description: Helpline for both sufferers and carers of people with phobias obsessional compulsive disorder, general anxieties, panic attacks, anorexia and bulimia, trauma withdrawal, also Telephone Self Help Groups, fact sheets, booklets, videos, audio tapes and books. We now offer help to carers of those who suffer borderline personality disorder.

Index keyword: Stress

Food and Chemical Allergy Association

27 Ferringham Lane
Ferring
West Sussex

Admin tel: 01903 241178

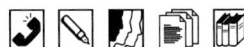

Description: Gives advice and practical guidance on how to discover and overcome allergies.

Index keyword: Allergies

Food Commission, The

94 White Lion Street
London
N1 9PF

Admin tel: 020 7837 2250
Admin fax: 020 7837 1141

Description: The Food Commission (UK) Ltd is a self-funded, independent consumer watchdog which campaigns for safer, healthier food.

Index keyword: Food

Foresight (The Association for the Promotion of Pre-Conceptual Care)

28 The Paddock
Godalming
Surrey
GU7 1XD

Helpline tel: **01483 427839**
Admin tel: 01483 427839
Admin fax: 01483 427668
Websight:
www.surreyweb.org.uk/foresight/home
Opening hours: usually 9.30am

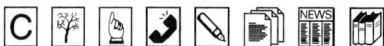

Description: Works to achieve healthy, normal babies by eliminating from parents' diet/environment/lifestyle factors known to cause fetal damage. This ensures that pregnancy starts with healthy sperm, ova and uterus.

Index keyword: Pregnancy and Childbirth

Forresters (National Schizophrenia Fellowship)

2 Southampton Road
Hythe
Hampshire
SO45 5GQ

Helpline tel: **01703 843042**
Admin tel: 01703 843042
Admin fax: 02380 841250

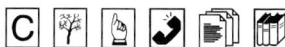

Description: A respite centre, providing breaks of up to one month for people with mental health problems or their carers. Offers several 'special weeks', including arts week, women's week, ethnic minorities week, young persons' weeks and carers' weeks.

Index keyword: Schizophrenia

Foundation for AIDS Counselling Treatment and Support (FACTS)

Between 23–25 Weston Park
Crouch End
London
N8 9SY

Admin tel: 020 8348 9195
Admin fax: 020 8340 5864

Description: Provides a wide range of high quality services, both medical and non-medical, to people affected by HIV/AIDS.

Index keyword: AIDS and HIV

Foundation for the Study of Infant Deaths, The

Artillery House
11–19 Artillery Row
London
SW1P 1RT

Helpline tel: **020 7233 2090**
Admin tel: 020 7222 8001
Admin fax: 020 7222 8002

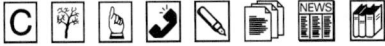

[icons]

Description: Works to prevent sudden infant death and promote infant health. FSID raises funds for research, gives support to families and provides information about infant death and infant care to families, health professionals and students.

Index keyword: Children: General Information

Freedom Organisation for the Right to Enjoy Smoking Tobacco (FOREST)

Audley House
13 Palace Street
London
SW12 5HX

Helpline tel: **07071 766537**
Admin fax: 020 7233 6144
Admin fax: 020 7630 6226

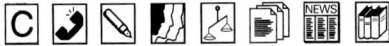

[icons]

Description: FOREST promotes equal rights for smokers and greater tolerance between smokers and non-smokers. It defends freedom of choice for adults who wish to smoke tobacco. It seeks to protect the rights of people wanting to make provision for smokers on their premises, from the encroachment of discriminating and persecutory legislation.

Index keyword: Smoking

FSH–MD Support Group (Muscular Dystrophy)

8 Caldecote Gardens
Bushy Heath
Herts
WD2 3RA

Admin tel: 020 8950 7500
Admin fax: 020 8950 7300
Website: www.btinternet.com/~fsh

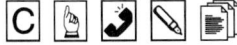

[icons]

Description: Offers support to sufferers and their carers; puts them in touch with members in their area. Arranges an annual informal get-together.

Index keyword: Muscular Dystrophy

FYD (Friends for Young Deaf People)

SE Embassy
East Court Mansion
College Lane
East Grinstead
RH19 3LT

Helpline tel: **01342 300080; 01342 324164 (minicom)**
Admin tel: 01342 300080
Admin fax: 01342 410232

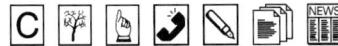

[icons]

Description: Promotes partnership between deaf and hearing people, to enable young deaf people to develop and become active members of society.

Index keyword: Hearing Problems/Deafness

G

Gamcare

25–27 Catherine Place
London
SW1E 6DU

Helpline: **0845 6000 133; Mon–Fri, 10.00am–10.00pm**
Admin tel: 020 7233 8988

Admin fax: 020 7233 8977
Website: www.gamcare.org.uk
E-mail: director@gamcare.org.uk

Description: This is a central point for information, advice and practical help on issues of people and gambling/electronic game playing. There is a national network of members. Telephone advice and counselling is provided for problem gamblers and their families.

Gardeners' Royal Benevolent Society, The

Bridge House
139 Kingston Road
Leatherhead
Surrey
KT22 7NT

Helpline tel: **01372 373962**
Admin tel: 01372 373962
Admin fax: 01372 362575

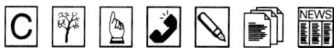

Description: Assists retired professional gardeners and their spouses with regular beneficiary payments and grants, and offers accommodation – sheltered, residential and nursing.

Index keyword: General Information

Gardening for the Disabled

Hayes Farm House
Hayes Lane
Peasmarsh
East Sussex
TN31 6XR

Admin tel: 01424 882876
Admin fax: 01424 882876

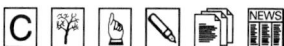

Description: Helps disabled people to take an active interest in gardening.

Index keyword: Gardening

Gauchers Association

25 West Cottages
London
NW6 1RJ

Helpline tel: **020 7433 1121**
Admin tel: 020 7433 1121
Website: www.gaucher.org.uk
E-mail: office@gaucher.net

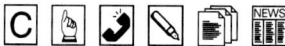

Description: Provides information about Gauchers disease and keeps families and medical advisers up to date with latest developments. Encourages the availability of treatment. Gauchers disease is an inherited enzyme-deficiency disorder.

Index keyword: Gaucher's Disease

General Council and Register of Naturopaths

Goswell House
2 Goswell Road
Street
Somerset
BA16 0JG

Helpline tel: **01458 840072**
Admin tel: 01458 840072
Admin fax: 01458 840075

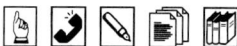

Description: The GCRN maintains a register of suitably qualified naturopaths, monitors educational standards in naturopathy and provides a code of professional conduct for its members, for the benefit and protection of the public.

Index keyword: Complementary Medicine

Genetic Interest Group

Unit 4D
Leroy House
436 Essex Road
London
N1 3QP

Helpline tel: **020 7430 0090**
Admin tel: 020 7704 3141
Admin fax: 020 7359 1447

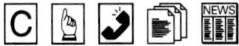

Description: GIG is the national alliance for voluntary groups supporting families with genetic disorders. It exists to raise awareness, to provide training for lay and professional people, to combat discrimination and to promote the development of appropriate, high quality services for people in need.

Index keyword: Genetics

Gideons International, The

Western House
George Street
Lutterworth
Leicestershire
LE17 4EE

Admin tel: 01455 554241
Admin fax: 01455 558267
Website: www.gideons.org.uk
E-mail: hq@gideons.org.uk
Opening times: 9.00am–5.15pm

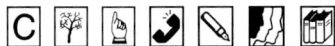

Description: Provides a free copy of the New Testament and Psalms to each hospital bed.

Index keyword: General Information

Gifted Children's Information Centre

Hampton Grange
21 Hampton Lane
Solihull
B91 2QJ

Helpline tel: **0121 705 4547**
Admin tel: 0121 705 4547
Admin fax: 0121 705 4547

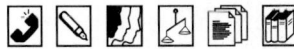

Description: Arranges psychological assessments and offers legal advice and guidance for children with special educational needs. Supplies books, guides, teaching packs and equipment for gifted children, dyslexic children and left-handed children.

Index keyword: Gifted Children

Gingerbread

16–17 Clerkenwell Close
London
EC1R 0AN

Helpline tel: **020 7336 8184**
Admin tel: 020 7336 8183
Admin fax: 020 7336 8185
Website: www.gingerbread.org.uk
E-mail: office@gingerbread.org.uk

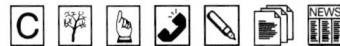

Description: Provides a network of self-help support groups for single parents and their children.

Index keyword: Childcare

Grandma's

PO Box 1392
London
SW6 4EJ

Admin tel: 020 7610 3904
Admin fax: 020 7610 3428
E-mail: grandmas@btinternet.com

Description: Grandma's is a church-based organisation which aims to provide practical help and support to children and families affected by HIV/AIDS. The services include baby-sitting, spending time with children after school or nursery, support with hospital appointments and outings for children.

Index keyword: AIDS and HIV

Great Britain Wheelchair Basketball Association

104 London Road
Chatteris
Cambridgeshire
PE16 6SF

Admin tel: 01354 695560
Admin fax: 01354 695752
E-mail: s.spika@gbwba.org.uk
Website: www.gbwba.org.uk

Description: Works for the promotion, development and organisation of wheelchair basketball in Great Britain. They have 65 teams playing basketball at different levels, from development leagues to European championships and Paralympics.

Index keyword: Disability: Sport/ Excercise

Group Against Steroid Prescriptions (GASP)

72 Costa Street
South Bank
Middlesbrough
Cleveland
TS6 6EU

Helpline tel: 01642 465118 (north); 01252 540033 (south)
Admin tel: 01642 465118
Admin tel: 01642 465118

Description: Aims to help and advise steroid patients suffering from adverse effects of the drugs. They have over 15,000 members around the UK.

Index keyword: Steroids

Guide Dogs for the Blind Association

Lanesborough House
15 Sandown Park South
Belfast
BT5 6HE

Admin tel: 02890 471453
Admin fax: 02890 655097
Website: www.gdba.org.uk
E-mail: belfast@gdba.org.uk

Description: Guide Dogs for the Blind is a voluntary organisation which aims to help visually impaired people to achieve greater levels of independence. This can be in the form of practical help, by the provision of a guide dog, rehabilitation training or information and advice on available services.

Index keyword: Blindness/Visual Handicap

Guide Dogs for the Blind Association, The

Hillfields
Burghfield Common
Reading
RG7 3YG

Helpline tel: 0118 9835555
Admin fax: 0118 9835433

Description: Breeds, trains and provides guide dogs. Training visually impaired people to use them safely. Other services and facilities for visually impaired people.

Index keyword: Blindness/Visual Handicap

Guideposts Trust Limited

Two Rivers
Station Lane
Witney
Oxon
OX8 6BH

Admin tel: 01993 772886
Admin fax: 01993 778160

C ⚘ ☝

Description: Provides day care services for people with mental health problems/learning disabilities; establishing a teaching nursing home for older mentally and physically frail people; recruits volunteers for befriending support; works in co-operation with statutory and voluntary agencies; raises charitable income to develop its projects.

Index keyword: Mental Health/Illness

Guild of Psychotherapists, The

19B Thornton Hill
London
SW19 4HU

Helpline tel: 0208 5404454
Admin tel: 0208 5404454
Admin fax: 0208 5404454
Opening times: Tues, Wed, Thurs 10am–1pm

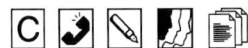

C ☎ ✎ 👣 📑

Description: Promotes, through psychotherapy offered by its members, the relief of psychological disturbance or disorder. Aims to provide a minimum four-year training in psychoanalytic psychotherapy, leading to UKCP registration.

Index keyword: Psychotherapy

Guillain–Barré Syndrome Support Group of the United Kingdom

Lincolnshire County Council Offices
Eastgate
Sleaford
Lincolnshire
NG34 7EB

Helpline tel: 0800 374803
Admin tel: 01529 304615
Admin fax: 01529 304615
Opening times: 24 hours

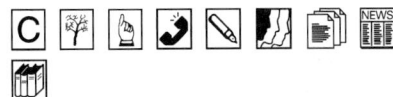

C ⚘ ☝ ☎ ✎ 👣 📑 NEWS 📖

Description: Provides emotional support to patients, relatives and friends and where possible personal visits by former patients. Educates and maintains awareness about the illness and the support group. Literature is available for the medical profession, patients and families. Supports research into the causes and treatment of the illness and encourages local and special interest groups.

Index keyword: Guillain–Barré Syndrome

H

Haemochromatosis Society

Holly Bush House
Hadley Green Road
Barnet
Hertfordshire
EN5 5PR

Helpline tel: 020 8449 1363
Admin tel: 020 8449 1363
Admin fax: 020 8449 1363
Website: www.ghsoc.org
E-mail: ghsoc@compuserve.com

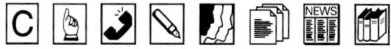

Description: Provides support and information to people with genetic haemochromatosis; encouragement to have their family members tested; and opportunities to contact others. Promotes awareness of this under-diagnosed common disorder – treatment is simple and effective – and encourages research.

Index keyword: Haemochromatosis

Haemophilia Society, The

3rd Floor
Chesterfield House
385 Euston Road
London
NW1 3AU

Helpline: **0800 0186068**
Admin tel: 020 7380 0600
Admin fax: 020 7387 8220
Website: www.haemophilia.org.uk
E-mail: info@haemophilia.org.uk
Opening times: 9.00am–5.00pm

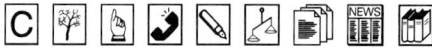

Description: Our mission is to ensure that people with haemophilia and other bleeding disorders receive the best possible treatment, care and support.

Index keyword: Haemophilia

Hairline International Alopecia Patients' Society (The)

Lyons Court
1668 High Street
Knowle
West Midlands
B93 0LY

Admin tel: 01564 775281
Admin fax: 01564 782270
Website: www.hairline.international.co.uk

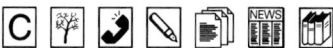

Description: Gives support and information to people experiencing alopecia and other types of hair loss. Meetings, newsletters and telephone advice. Enquirers should enclose A4 self-addressed envelope.

Index keyword: Hair

Half PINNT (for children)

Riverside Lodge
London Road
Whitehouses, Retford
Nottinghamshire
DN22 7JG

Helpline tel: **01777 710723**
Admin tel: 01777 710723
Admin fax: 01777 710723

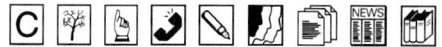

Description: Aims to help adults, children and families feed artificially. Provides support groups, local regional groups, quarterly magazine, equipment bank, school booklets, etc.

Index keyword: Children: General Information

HCPT, The Pilgrimage Trust

100a High Street
Banstead
Surrey
SM7 2RB

Helpline tel: **01737 353311**
Admin fax: 01737 353008
Website: www.hcpt.org.uk
E-mail: hq@hcpt.org.uk

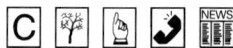

Description: Takes people to Lourdes, especially those suffering from illness or disability.

Index keyword: Disability: Care Scheme/ Holidays

Harry Edwards Spiritual Healing Sanctuary Trust, The

Burrows Lea
Shere
Guildford
Surrey
GU5 9QG

Helpline tel: **01483 202054**
Admin tel: 01483 202054
Website:
ds.dial.pipex.com/town/parade/na72

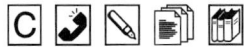

Description: The Harry Edwards Spiritual Healing Sanctuary exists to help those who are sick or suffering in any way, through absent (distant) or contact healing. The administrators also hold healing seminars, give healing demonstrations and lectures and welcome visiting groups to the Sanctuary.

Index keyword: Complementary Medicine

Headway: Brain Injury Association

4 King Edward Court
King Edward Street
Nottingham
NG1 1EW

Helpline tel: **0115 924 0800**
Admin tel: 0115 924 0800
Admin fax: 0115 958 4446
Website: www.headway.org.uk
E-mail: enquiries@headway.org.uk

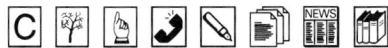

Description: Aims to promote understanding of all aspects of head injury and to provide information, support and services to people with head injury, their families and carers.

Index keyword: Head Injury

Health Information Wales

Health Promotion Division
Ffynnon-las
Ty Glas Avenue, Llanishen
Cardiff
CF14 5EZ

Helpline tel: **01792 776252**
Admin tel: 029 2075 2222
Admin fax: 029 2075 6000
Website: www.hpw.wales.gov.uk
Opening hours: 9.00am–5.00pm

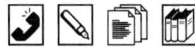

Description: Health Information Wales is a national health information service run by Health Promotion Wales on behalf of the Welsh Assembly. It forms part of the Patient's Charter initiative and provides free, confidential information to the public and health professionals in Wales.

Index keyword: Patients Rights

Health Service Ombudsman for England

Millbank Tower
Millbank
London
SW1P 4QP

Helpline tel: **020 7217 4051**
Admin tel: 020 7276 3000
Admin fax: 020 7217 4940

Description: Investigates complaints about the NHS when the complainant remains dissatisfied following the investigation of the complaint by the local hospital, clinic or surgery.

Index keyword: Ombudsman

H

Healthline Health Information Service

St Margaret's House
21 Old Ford Road
London
E2 9PL

Helpline tel: **0800 665544**
Admin tel: 020 8983 1225
Admin fax: 020 8983 1553
E-mail: info@tcoh.demon.co.uk
Opening hours: 9.00am–7.00pm, Mon–Thurs; 9.00am–5.00pm, Fri.

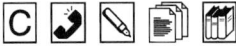

Description: Provides a health information service, covering local services, self-help groups, waiting times and charter standards.

Index keyword: General Health

Healthpoint

Freepost BM 3007
Dudley
DY2 8BR

Helpline tel: **0800 665544**
Admin tel: 01384 215555
Admin fax: 01384 215559

Description: Healthpoint provides information on all aspects of Health services, conditions and diseases, self-help, waiting times, complaints procedures, patient's charter, health improvement and community care. This is part of NHS Direct.

Index keyword: Patients Rights

Healthwise Helpline

First Floor
Cavern Court
8 Mathew Street
Liverpool
L2 6RE

Helpline tel: **0800 665544**
Admin tel: 0151 227 4150
Admin fax: 0151 227 4019
Website: www.healthwise.org.uk
E-mail: admin@healthwise.org.uk
Opening times: Every day 9am–9pm

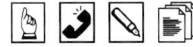

Description: Healthwise is a health information and promotion service. The project is managed by a private company, Healthwise Helpline Ltd. Healthwise is contracted to the North West Regional Health Authority to provide health information services to Merseyside, Cheshire, Lancashire, Greater Manchester, South Cumbria and Glossop, Cambridgeshire region and Cambridgeshire Health Authority.

Index keyword: General Health

Hearing Dogs for the Deaf

The Training Centre
London Road (A40)
Lewknor
Oxon
OX49 5RY

Helpline tel: **01844 353898**
Admin tel: 01844 353898
Admin fax: 01844 353099

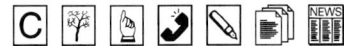

Description: Trains dogs to act as ears of severely or profoundly deaf people. The dog is taught to respond to household sounds (doorbell, smoke alarm, baby crying) by finding its deaf owner, alerting by touch and leading back to the sound. No charge is made to recipients.

Index keyword: Hearing Problems/ Deafness

Hearing Research Trust

330–332 Gray's Inn Road
London
WC1X 8EE

Helpline tel: **020 7833 1733**
Admin tel: 020 7833 1733
Admin fax: 020 7278 0404

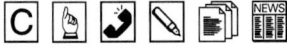

C ✋ 📞 ✏️ 📑 📰

Description: The trust is a charity dedicated to improving the lives of deaf and hard of hearing people through research. Priority areas include glue ear, detecting deafness in babies, inherited deafness, hearing aids, tinnitus and repair of damage to the inner ear.

Index keyword: Hearing Problems/ Deafness

Help for Health Trust (Health Information Service)

Highcroft
Romsey Road
Winchester
Hampshire
SO22 5DH

Helpline tel: **0800 665544**
Admin tel: 01962 849100
Admin fax: 01962 849079

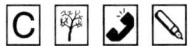

C 🌳 📞 ✏️

Description: The Health Information Service is a network of NHS funded helplines linked to a single national freephone number. Information is available on selfhelp groups, NHS services, illnesses and treatments, waiting times and patients rights.

Index keyword: General Information

Help The Aged

16–18 St James's Walk
London
EC1R 0BE

Helpline tel: **0808 8006565**
Admin tel: 020 7253 0253
Admin fax: 020 7251 0747
Website: www.helptheaged.org.uk
E-mail: info@helptheaged.org.uk

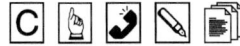

C ✋ 📞 ✏️ 📑

Description: Works to improve the quality of life of older people, particularly those who are frail, isolated or poor. Runs Seniorline a freephone advice service for senior citizens, their relatives and carers – call see separate entry. Help the Aged also provides a range of free advice leaflets covering many matters: housing, home safety and health.

Index keyword: Elderly: General Information

Help The Aged (Northern Ireland)

Ascot House
Shaftesbury Square
Belfast
BT2 7DB

Helpline tel: **0808 8006565**
Admin tel: 02890 230666
Admin fax: 02890 248183
E-mail: claire.killen@helptheaged.org.uk

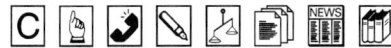

C ✋ 📞 ✏️ 🔺 📑 📰 📖

Description: Help The Aged provides practical support to help older people live independent lives, particularly those who are frail, isolated or poor.

Index keyword: Elderly: General Information

Hemi-Help

Bedford House
215 Balham High Road
London
SW17 7BQ

Admin tel: 020 87670210
Admin fax: 020 87670319

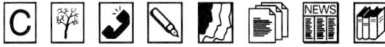

[icons]

Description: Provides information and support for children with hemiplegia.

Index keyword: Disability: Children

Herpes Viruses Association

41 North Road
London
N7 9DP

Helpline tel: **020 7609 9061**
Admin tel: 020 7607 9661
Website: www.herpes.org.uk

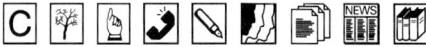

[icons]

Description: Gives accurate information to public, media and health professionals on the herpes simplex virus. Provides counselling and advice for people affected physically or psychologically.

Index keyword: Herpes

HME Contact Group

3 Linn Drive
Netherlee
Glasgow
G44 3PT

Helpline tel: **0141 633 2617**
E-mail:
hmecontactgropup@tinyworld.co.uk

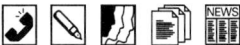

[icons]

Description: Provides a point of contact for parents and carers of children with HME, usually just after diagnosis, to share experiences or just talk. The group also offers some literature on the condition.

Index keyword: Children: General Information

Holiday Care

2nd Floor
Imperial Building
Victoria Road
Horley
RH6 7PZ

Helpline tel: **01293 774535**
Admin tel: 01293 771500
Admin fax: 01293 784647
Website:
www.freespace.virgin.net/hol.care
E-mail: holiday.care@virgin.net

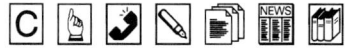

[icons]

Description: Holiday Care is the UK's central source of information and support for disabled and disadvantaged people wishing to take a holiday.

Index keyword: Disability: Care Scheme/ Holidays

Holiday Endeavour for Lone Parents (HELP)

57 Owston Road
Carcroft
Doncaster
DN6 7NY

Admin tel: 01302 726959
Admin fax: 01302 726959

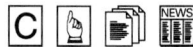

[icons]

Description: The charity aims to provide good quality, low cost holidays for lone parent families.

Index keyword: Holidays

Holistic Resources Limited

Cribden House
Rossendale Hospital
Rossendale
Lancashire
BB4 6NE

Helpline tel: **01706 240080**
Admin tel: 01706 240083
Admin fax: 01706 240082
E-mail: rossendalhospice@airtime.co.uk

Description: Aims to make available an effective treatment for sufferers of irritable bowel syndrome and other gut disorders.

Index keyword: Holistic

Home Library Service

Central Library
Clapham Road South
Lowestoft
Suffolk
NR32 1DR

Admin tel: 01502 405338
Admin fax: 01502 405350

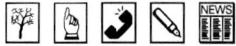

Description: The Home Library Service is available to any person who is unable to visit the nearest local library or mobile library because of age, handicap or illness. Library visits are usually on a fortnightly basis and are free of charge.

Index keyword: Disability: General Information

Home-Start UK

2 Salisbury Road
Leicester
LE1 7QR

Helpline tel: **0116 233 9955**
Admin tel: 0116 233 9955
Admin fax: 0116 233 0232
Website: www.home-start.org.uk
E-mail: info@home-start.org.uk

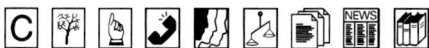

Description: Home-Start is a voluntary organisation with branches throughout the UK, offering support, friendship and practical help at home to families with pre-school children experiencing difficulties and stress. Volunteers, who are parents themselves, visit families in their own homes, helping to prevent family crisis and breakdown.

Index keyword: Family Support and Welfare

Homoeopathic Trust, The

Hahnemann House
2 Powis Place
Great Ormond Street
London
WC1N 3HT

Helpline tel: **020 7837 9469**
Admin tel: 020 7837 9469
Admin fax: 020 7278 7900

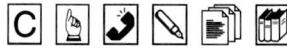

Description: The Trust (incorporating The Homoeopathic Society) is committed to the promotion and development of homoeopathy. Provides information on homoeopathy and publishes a list of registered doctors trained in homoeopathic medicine.

Index keyword: Complementary Medicine

Hope UK

25f Copperfield Street
London
SE1 0EN

Helpline tel: **020 7928 0848**
Admin tel: 020 7928 0848
Admin fax: 020 7401 3477
Website: www.hopeuk.org
E-mail: hope@hopeuk.org

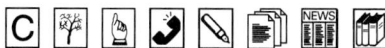

Description: Provides alcohol and drug prevention education for children and young people, supplies high quality resources, training, speakers, parents' programmes, as reduce alcohol and other drug-related problems.

Index keyword: Alcohol Problems

Horder Centre for Arthritis, The

St Johns Road
Crowborough
East Sussex
TN6 1XP

Admin tel: 01892 665577
Admin fax: 01892 662142
Opening times: 9am–5pm

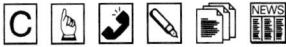

[icons: C, hand, phone, pencil, documents, NEWS]

Description: Aims to provide professional help by all available methods for people suffering the pain and disabling effects of all forms of arthritis; to restore maximum independence and alleviate pain, wherever possible; as a centre of excellence, to remain at the forefront of the battle against arthritis.

Index keyword: Arthritis/Rheumatic Disorders

Hospice Information Service

St Christopher's Hospice
51 Lawrie Park Road
London
SE26 6DZ

Helpline tel: 020 8778 9252
Admin tel: 020 8778 9252
Admin fax: 020 8776 9345
Website: www.hospiceinformation.co.uk
E-mail: info@his2.freeserve.co.uk

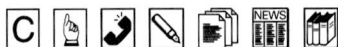

[icons: C, hand, phone, pencil, documents, NEWS, book]

Description: Acts as worldwide link between those involved in palliative care.

Maintains directories of hospices in the UK and overseas. Enquiries welcomed from public and professionals.

Index keyword: Hospice

Housing Organisations Mobility and Exchange Service (HOMES)

26 Chapter Street
London
SW1P 4ND

Admin tel: 020 7233 7077
Admin fax: 020 7976 6947

[icons: phone, pencil, documents]

Description: HOMES is responsible for promoting opportunities for mobility in the public and social housing sectors through HOMESWAP and the HOMES Mobility Scheme. Over 45,000 tenants are registered on HOMESWAP. Updated lists of tenants who want to swap homes are issued monthly to local authorities.

Index keyword: Housing

Human Fertilisation and Embryology Authority

Paxton House
30 Artillery Lane
London
E1 7LS

Admin tel: 020 7377 5077
Admin fax: 020 7377 1871
Website: www.hfea.gov.uk

[icons: pencil, documents]

Description: The HFEA regulates and licenses fertility clinics offering in vitro fertilisation and donor insemination. Patients can be provided with information about these treatments.

Index keyword: Infertility

Human Rights Society

Mariners Hard
Cley
Nr Holt
Norfolk
NR25 7RX

Helpline tel: **01263 740990**
Admin tel: 01263 740990
Admin fax: 01263 740990

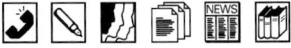

Description: Opposes the legalisation of voluntary euthanasia, because they can see no way in which any law could provide the necessary safeguards. Educational material and information on pain relief and hospice care are provided.

Index keyword: Euthanasia

Hyperactive Children's Support Group

71 Whyke Lane
Chichester
West Sussex
PO19 2LD

Admin tel: 01903 725182
Admin fax: 01903 734726
Website: www.hyperactive.force9.co.uk
E-mail: hacsg@hyperactive.force9.co.uk

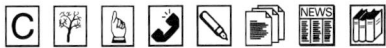

Description: Aims to help and support hyperactive children and their parents; to conduct research and promote investigation into the incidence of hyperactivity in the UK, its causes and treatments; and to disseminate information concerning this condition.

Index keyword: Hyperactive Children

IA (The Ileostomy and Internal Pouch Support Group)

PO Box 123
Scunthorpe
DN15 9YW

Helpline tel: **0800 0184724**
Admin fax: 01724 721601

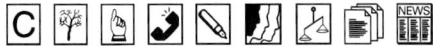

Description: The Ileostomy and Internal Pouch Support Group formed the Ileostomy Association. IA is a mutual aid association whose aim is to help people who have had their colon removed to return to a fully active and normal life as soon as possible, IA works closely with with the medical profession, the manufacturers and others, IA also supports research into casual illnesses and ways of improving the quality of life with an ileostomy.

Index keyword: Digestive Problems

Immunity Legal Centre

1st Floor
32–38 Osnaburgh Street
London
NW1 3ND

Helpline tel: **020 7388 6776**
Admin tel: 020 7388 6776
Admin fax: 020 7388 6371

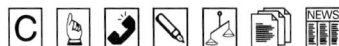

Description: Provides free and confidential legal advice, information and representation to anyone with, or affected by, HIV or AIDS.

Index keyword: AIDS and HIV

Impotence Information Centre

PO Box 1130
London
W3 OBB

Description: Provides information on the treatment of male erectile dysfunction (impotence).

Index keyword: Impotence

Impotence World Service (IWS)

119 South Ruth Street
Maryville
USA
TN 37803

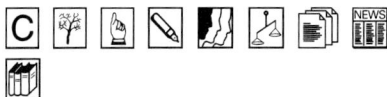

Description: Self-help groups similar to Alcoholics Anonymous and Al-Anon. They have Impotence Anonymous (IA) and I-Anon (for partners) chapters. Publications available.

Index keyword: Impotence

In Touch

10 Norman Road
Sale
Cheshire
M33 3DF

Admin tel: 0161 905 2440
Admin fax: 0161 718 5787
E-mail:
worthington@netscapeonline.co.uk

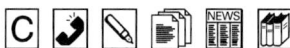

Description: In Touch is an information and contact service for parents of children with special needs. Especially rare disorders.

Index keyword: Disability: Children

In Touch Publishing

37 Charles Street
Cardiff
CF1 4EB

Admin tel: 029 2022 2403
Admin fax: 029 2022 2383

Description: The *In Touch Handbook* is the essential guide to visual impairment and is packed with information about equipment, services and advice for visually impaired people. The *In Touch Care Guide* series provides some concise, practical advice on specific areas of visual impairment.

Index keyword: Blindness/Visual Handicap

Incontact

United House
North Road
London
N7 9DP

Helpline tel: 020 7700 7035
Admin fax: 020 7700 7045
Website: www.incontact.org
E-mail: edu@incontact.org

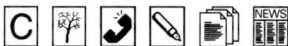

Description: Incontact is a membership organisation for people with bladder or bowel problems. It offers information, advice and support, including a quarterly newsletter written by people who know

THE HEALTH ADDRESS BOOK 2000–2001: A Directory of Health Support Groups

what it's like to have a bladder or bowel condition. It also tests new products and provides speakers for the media.

Index keyword: Digestive Problems

Independent Adoption Service

121–123 Camberwell Road
London
SE5 OHB

Admin tel: 020 7703 1088
Admin fax: 020 7277 1668
Website:
www.independentadoptionservice.org.uk

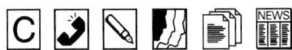

Description: Independent Adoption Service is a small approved voluntary adoption agency. It specialises in finding families for children from the care system who are unable to be brought up within their own families.

Index keyword: Adoption and Fostering

Independent Care After Incestuous Relationship and Rape

Gate House
Whiteways
Greater Chesterford
Essex
CB10 1NX

Helpline tel: **01799 530520 (Answering machine out of hours)**
Admin tel: 01799 530520
Opening times: 9am–5pm

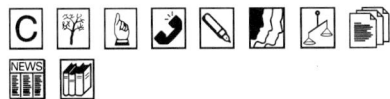

Description: To facilitate a survivors recovery from the complete legacy of

child/sexual abuse. Celebrates National Incest Awareness Day (annually) 2 April. Participates in the Prevention of Child Abuse *Bridgework* telephone support.

Index keyword: Rape/Battered Women

Independent Healthcare Association

22 Little Russell Street
London
WC 1A 2HT

Admin tel: 020 7430 0537
Admin fax: 020 7242 2681
Website: www.iha.org.uk

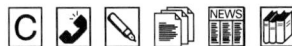

Description: Aims to promote and protect standards of healthcare in the independent sector.

Index keyword: General Health

Independent Living 93 Fund

PO Box 183
Nottingham
NG8 3RD

Helpline tel: **0115 942 8191**
Admin tel: 0115 942 8192
Admin fax: 0115 929 3156

Description: This government-funded trust provides cash payments to severely disabled people within the community, enabling them to pay for extra care to supplement that provided by the local authority.

Index keyword: Disability: General Information

Information Service on Disability

Oak Tree Lane Centre
91 Oak Tree Lane
Selly Oak
Birmingham
B29 6JA

Helpline tel: **0121 414 1495**
Admin tel: 0121 627 1627 ext 53252
Admin fax: 0121 627 8210

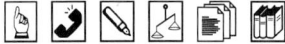

Description: An information service providing help and advice on a wide range of disability-related issues. Advice is free, confidential and impartial. Also have a wide range of information, available in different forms: books, leaflets, magazines, videos, tapes and braille.

Index keyword: Disability: General Information

Informed Parent, The

19 Woodlands Road
Harrow
Middlesex
HA1 2RT

Helpline tel: **020 8861 1022**
Admin tel: 020 8861 1022
Admin fax: 020 8861 1022

Description: Promotes awareness and understanding about vaccination, in order to preserve the freedom of an informed choice. Offers support to parents, regardless of the decisions they make.

Index keyword: General Information

Institute for Complementary Medicine

PO Box 194
London
SE16 1QZ

Helpline tel: **020 7237 5165**
Admin tel: 020 7237 5175

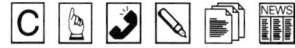

Description: Offers names of complementary practitioners and lists of teaching organisations in complementary medicine. Also offers information for the media on the whole field of complementary medicine.

Index keyword: Complementary Medicine

Institute for Optimum Nutrition, The (ION)

Blades Court
Deodar Road
London
SW15 2NU

Admin tel: 020 8877 9993
Admin fax: 020 8877 9980
Website: www.ion.ac.uk
E-mail: info@ion.ac.uk

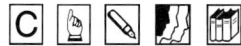

Description: ION is an independent educational trust which helps people achieve optimum nutrition and aim for the highest level of health.

Index keyword: Nutrition/Diet

Institute of Electrolysis

PO Box 5187
Milton Keynes
MK4 2ZF

Helpline tel: **01908 521511**
Admin tel: 01908 695297

Admin fax: 01908 695297
Website: www.electrolysis.co.uk
E-mail: institute@electrolysis.co.uk

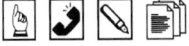

Description: The Institute of Electrolysis is a non-profit making organisation established in 1944. It is a central representative body for electrologists and its activities embrace every aspect of the profession.

Index keyword: Complementary Medicine

Insulin Dependent Diabetes Trust

PO Box 294
Northampton
NN1 4XS

Helpline tel: **01604 622837**
Admin tel: 01604 622837
Admin fax: 01604 622838
Website: www.iddtinternational.org
E-mail: enquiries@iddtinternational.org

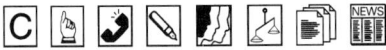

Description: The trust helps and supports people living with diabetes, especially people experiencing problems with genetically produced human insulin. The trust ensures that all people with diabetes have an informed choice of treatment and tries to ensure that animal insulin continues to be available for people who need it.

Index keyword: Diabetes

International Autistic Research Organisation, The (Autism Research Limited)

49 Orchard Avenue
Shirley
Croydon
CRO 7NE

Helpline tel: **020 8777 0095**
Admin tel: 020 8777 0095
Admin fax: 020 8776 2362
E-mail: iaro@lineone.net

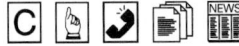

Description: Information, provision and awareness raising of scientific research into Autism.

Index keyword: Autism

International College of Oriental Medicine (UK) Limited, The

Green Hedges House
Green Hedges Avenue
East Grinstead
West Sussex
RH19 1DZ

Helpline tel: **01342 313106**
Admin tel: 01342 313107
Admin fax: 01342 318302
Website: www.orientalmed.ac.uk
E-mail: admin@orientalmed.ac.uk

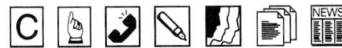

Description: Promotes healing and the maintenance of good health through the use of acupuncture and therapeutic massage. Training courses in acupuncture and therapeutic massage also available.

Index keyword: Complementary Medicine

International Federation of Reflexologists

76–78 Edridge Road
Croydon
Surrey
CRO 1EF

Helpline tel: **020 8667 9458**
Admin tel: 020 8667 9458
Admin fax: 020 8649 9291
Website: www.ifr44@aol.com
Opening times: 9.30am–5.00pm

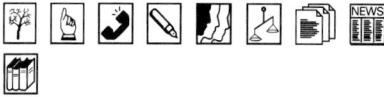

Description: The Federation was formed in the 1980s by a group of professional reflexologists, who felt that training standards and levels of professional competence were not high enough. The Federation has hundreds of members all over the world, bound by a strict code of ethics and practice. It has a list of professional therapists and accredited schools.

Index keyword: Complementary Medicine

International Glaucoma Association

108c Warner Road
Camberwell
London
SE5 9HQ

Helpline tel: **020 7737 3265**
Admin tel: 020 7737 3265
Admin fax: 020 7346 5929
Website: www.iga.org.uk/home.htm
E-mail: info@iga.org.uk

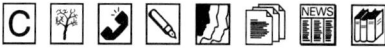

Description: The IGA aims to prevent loss of sight from glaucoma throughout the world. Membership is worldwide and open to patients and interested professionals. Patient information is provided free of charge. Also supports research into glaucoma and its treatment.

Index keyword: Eye Care

International Planned Parenthood Federation

Regent's College
Inner Circle
Regent's Park
London
NW3 4NS

Admin tel: 020 7486 7900
Admin fax: 020 7487 7950

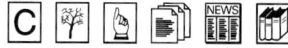

Description: The IPPF, founded in 1952, is the world's leading voluntary family healthcare organisation, working on a global scale to promote and provide sexual and reproductive health and family planning services, and to develop public support for sustainable population, environment and development policies.

Index keyword: Family Planning

International Society of Professional Aromatherapists

ISPA House
82 Ashby Road
Hinckley
Leicestershire
LE10 1SN

Helpline tel: **01455 637987**
Admin tel: 01455 637987
Admin fax: 01455 890956
E-mail: lisabrown@ispa.demon.co.uk

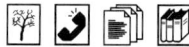

Description: This is the largest association of aromatherapists, offering professional credibility to its members and accredited courses to trainees. It aims to maintain and develop high standards of qualification and practice within the membership and throughout the profession as a whole. It provides a quarterly journal, annual conference, members' register, free lists of local therapists and general information.

Index keyword: Complementary Medicine

International Spinal Research Trust

100 Crossbrook Street
Cheshunt
Hertfordshire
EN8 8JJ

Helpline tel: **01992 641999**
Admin fax: 01992 640641

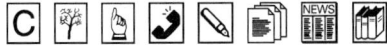

C ⚘ 👆 📞 ✏ 🗐 NEWS 📖

Description: ISRT exists to fund research, on an international level, with the sole aim of ending the permanence of paralysis caused by spinal cord injury.

Index keyword: Spinal Injuries

International Stress Management Association

PO Box 348
Waltham Cross
London
EN8 8ZL

Admin tel: 07000 780 430
E-mail: stress@isma.org.uk
Website: www.isma.org.uk

C 👆

Description: ISMA (UK) is the professional association for people whose work centres on stress management. It exists for the spread of sound knowledge, the maintenance of quality and to resource its members. Activities include an annual conference, forum or debate and validating stress management trainers. ISMA provides a referral service to put those in need in touch with service providers. Contact is preferred in writing or by e-mail.

Index keyword: Stress

Interstitial Cystitis Support Group

76 High Street
Stony Stratford
Bucks
MK11 iAH

Admin tel: 01908 569169
Admin fax: 01908 569169
Website: www.interstitialcystitis.co.uk
E-mail: info@interstitialcystitis.co.uk

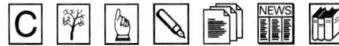

C ⚘ 👆 ✏ 🗐 NEWS 📖

Description: Works for the relief of sickness of persons suffering from interstitial cystitis. Provides patients, their families and friends with contact with other sufferers in their area. Promotes the advancement of education amongst the general public and the medical profession into the causes and treatments of IC.

Index keyword: Cystitis

Invalid Children's Aid Nationwide (I CAN)

4 Dyers Building
Holborn
London
EC1N 2QP

Admin tel: 0870 0104066
Admin fax: 0870 01040-67

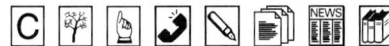

C ⚘ 👆 📞 ✏ 🗐 NEWS 📖

Description: Runs schools and nurseries for children with speech and language problems. Offers training courses and publications for professionals in speech and language.

Index keyword: Speech Difficulties

IPSEA

22 Warren Hill Road
Woodbridge
Suffolk
1P12 4DU

Helpline tel: 01394 382814
Admin tel: 01394 380518
Admin fax: 01394 380518

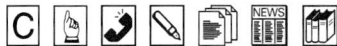

[C] [☚] [✆] [✎] [📄] [NEWS] [📖]

Description: Provides independent advice on local education authorities' legal duties towards children with special education needs.

Index keyword: Education

Irish Cancer Society

5 Northumberland Road
Dublin 4
Ireland

Helpline tel: 1800 200 700
Admin tel: 00 3531 668 1855
Admin fax: 00 3531 668 7599
E-mail: admin@irishcancer.ie

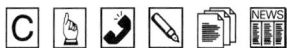

[C] [☚] [✆] [✎] [📄] [NEWS]

Description: Provides information, support and guidance for patients, families and professionals or anyone concerned about cancer. Services include cancer helpline, night nursing, daffodil funded home care nursery, support groups, practical help for patients, research and education.

Index keyword: Cancer

Irritable Bowel Syndrome Network (IBS Network)

St John's House
Hither Green Hospital
Hither Green Lane
London
SE13 6RU

Helpline tel: 020 8698 4611 ext 8194 (enquiries)
Admin tel: 020 8698 4611 ext 8194

Admin fax: 020 8698 5655
Opening times: Mon, Wed, Fri 10.30am–1.30pm

[C] [🌿] [☚] [✆] [✎] [📄] [NEWS]

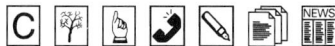

Description: The network is run for sufferers by sufferers, to help alleviate the distress and suffering associated with the condition.

Index keyword: Bowel

Issue (The National Fertility Association)

114 Litchfield Street
Walsall
West Midlands
WS1 1SZ

Helpline tel: 01922 722 888
Admin tel: 01922 722 888
Admin fax: 01922 640070
Website: www.issue.co.uk
E-mail: webmaster@issue.co.uk

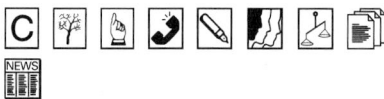

[C] [🌿] [☚] [✆] [✎] [👣] [⚖] [📄] [NEWS]

Description: Provides information, support and representation to people with fertility difficulties and to people who work with them.

Index keyword: Infertility

ITP Support Association

'Synehurste'
Kimbolton Road
Bolnhurst
Bedfordshire
MK44 2EW

Helpline tel: 01234 376559
Admin tel: 01234 376559
Admin fax: 01234 376559

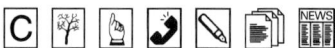

[C] [🌿] [☚] [✆] [✎] [📄] [NEWS]

Description: Aims to promote the general welfare of patients with ITP by providing patients support, advice on referrals, a telephone contact network with other sufferers, a fact sheet for schools with ITP pupils; to collate information and work with the medical profession to advance the knowledge and treatment of ITP.

Index keyword: General Information

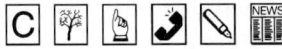

J

Jewish AIDS Trust

Walsingham House
1331–7 High Road
London
N20 9HR

Helpline tel: **020 8446 8228**
Admin fax: 020 8446 8227

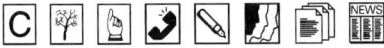

Description: Provides the Jewish community with education on HIV/ AIDS; offers face-to-face counselling and support to people infected or affected by HIV/AIDS.

Index keyword: AIDS and HIV

Jewish Blind and Disabled

"Fairacres"
164 East End Road
East Finchley
London
N2 0RR

Helpline tel: **020 8883 1000**
Admin fax: 020 8844 6729

Description: The society provides modern sheltered housing (self-contained flats) with communal facilities, amenities and welfare services for Jewish blind, partially-sighted and disabled persons, couples and families.

Index keyword: Disability: General Information

Jewish Care

221 Golders Green Road
Stuart Young House
Golders Green
London
NW11 9DQ

Helpline tel: **020 8922 2222**
Admin tel: 020 8922 2000
Admin fax: 020 8922 1998
E-mail: info@jcare.org
Opening times: 9.00am–5.30pm, Mon–Fri

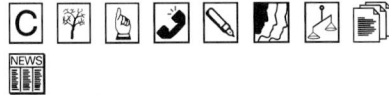

Description: Providing an unparaelled network of social services care provisions for Jewish people living in London and South East England. For elderly, mentally ill, physically disabled and blind people, as well as those who are unemployed, and Holocaust survivors.

Index keyword: Ethnic Minorities

Jewish Marriage Council

23 Ravenshurst Avenue
Hendon
London
NW4 4EE

Helpline tel: **020 8203 6311 (MIYAD)**
Admin tel: 020 8203 6311
Admin fax: 020 8203 8727
E-mail: jmc@dircon.co.uk

Opening times: 12.00am–12.00pm, Sun–Thur;
Fri–12.00am till one hour before Sabbath, Sat
from one hour after Sabbath untill midnight.

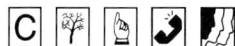

Description: JMC operated a crisis line
(MIYAD) as well as a counselling service,
groups for divorced & separated people,
self-esteem groups, pre-marriage education
groups, mediation for divorcing couples
and a Get (religiuos divorce) Advisory
Service. Also operates the Connect Jewish
Marriage Bureau (020 8203 5207).

Index keyword: Ethnic Minorities

Joint Committee on Mobility for Disabled People

Woodcliff House
51a Cliff Road
Weston-Super-Mare
Somerset
BS22 9SE

Helpline tel: **01934 642313**
Admin tel: 01934 642313

Description: Campaigns to improve
transport, access and mobility interests of
physically disabled people. Made up of 30
charities and voluntary and other
relevant organisations, it works in the
area of policy and is consulted by central
and local government and others.

Index keyword: Disability: General
Information

Joubert Syndrome Support Group

76–78 Coniston Avenue
Little Hulton
Worsley
M38 9WZ

Helpline tel: **0161 950 0749; 0161 799 2502**
Admin tel: 0161 950 0749

Description: This family run-organisation
offers support to other families who have
children with this rare syndrome. It
provides information and a chance to
talk. The Group also works to spread the
word about this condition and bring it to
the attention of more people, including
doctors and nurses.

Index keyword: Childcare

Justice Awareness Basic Support (JABS)

1 Gawsworth Road
Golborne
Nr Warrington
Cheshire
WA3 3RF

Helpline tel: **01942 713565**
Admin tel: 01942 713565
Admin fax: 01942 201323

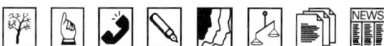

Description: JABS, as a self-help support
group, neither recommends nor advises
against vaccinations, but aims to promote
understanding about immunisations and
offer basic support to any parent whose
child has a health problem after
vaccination.

Index keyword: Childcare

THE HEALTH ADDRESS BOOK 2000–2001: A Directory of Health Support Groups

Justice for all Vaccine Damaged Children UK

Erin's Cottage
Fussells Building, Whiteway Road
St. George
Bristol
BS5 7QY

Helpline tel: **0117 955 7817**
Admin tel: 0117 955 7818
Opening times: Mon-Thurs 9am-9pm, Fri 12pm-9pm

Description: Offers an in touch service to parents of children damaged by vaccination. Deals with enquiries from Health Authorities, Social Services, Doctors and Solicitors and gives advice on when and how to claim, tribunal procedures etc.

Index keyword: Children: General Information

K

Keep Fit Association

Astra House
Suite 105
Acklow Road
London
SE14 6EE

Admin tel: 020 8692 9566
Admin fax: 020 8692 8383

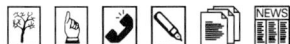

Description: KFA is a national

organisation supported by the Sports Council. It has 12,000 members and over 1,500 professionally qualified teachers, making it one of the largest and most effective fitness bodies in the UK.

Index keyword: General Health

Keratoconus Self-Help and Support Association

Po Box 26251
London
W3 9WQ

Helpline tel: **020 8692 9566**
Admin tel: 020 8692 8383

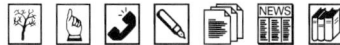

Description: Provides information and support for people affected by keratoconus and raises awareness of the condition among opticians and other professionals. Also raises money for research.

Index keyword: Eye Care

Kids Active

Pryor's Bank
Bishops Park
London
SW6 3LA

Helpline: **020 7731 1435**
Admin tel: 020 7736 4443
Admin fax: 020 7731 4426
Website: www.kidsactive.org.uk
E-mail: office@kidsactive.org.uk
Opening times: 9.00am–5.00pm

Kids' Clubs Network

Bellerive House
3 Muirfield Crescent
London
E14 9SZ

Helpline tel: 020 7512 2100
Admin tel: 020 7512 2112
Admin fax: 020 7512 2010

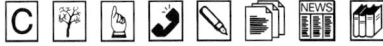

Description: This is the only national organisation working exclusively to promote and support childcare for school age children.

Index keyword: Childcare

Kidscape

2 Grosvenor Gardens
London
SW1W 0DH

Admin tel: 020 7730 3300
Admin fax: 020 7730 7081
Website: www.kidscape.org.uk
E-mail: contact@kidscape.org.uk
Opening times: 10.00am–4.00pm

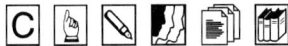

Description: Kidscape is a charity dedicated to keeping children safe. It is the only natio-wide charity committed to preventing child sexual abuse and bullying. We provide:

* A helpline offering advice and support for the parents of bullied children
* A Letter Network – a penpal service for bullied children
* A nation-wide training programme covering topics from anti-bullying to staff and interpersonal development
* Publishing books, videos, posters and free booklets and leaflets on ways to tackle both bullying and child abuse
* Conferences and research on bullying and child safety.

Index keyword: Childcare

King's Fund

11–13 Cavendish Square
London
W1G 0AN

Admin tel: 020 7307 2400
Admin fax: 020 7307 2801
Website: www.kingsfund.org.uk

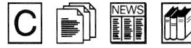

Description: The Fund aims to secure for Londoners, including the most vulnerable and deprived, the best possible health and health care; to stimulate and disseminate good practice and innovation in health and related services; to make an independent contribution to the development of health policy, nationally and internationally.

Index keyword: General Information

Kingston Women's Centre

169 Canbury Park Road
Kingston upon Thames
Surrey
KT2 6LG

Helpline tel: 020 8541 1964; 020 8541 1941

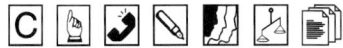

Description: Provides a service by and for women, which includes counselling (especially on sexual abuse); support; information on a range of topics, including legal advice on housing, relationship breakdown etc; and some stress-relieving complementary therapy. All therapists are properly trained and supervised where appropriate.

Index keyword: Women's Health

Kith and Kids

3rd Floor Irish Centre
Pretoria Road
Tottenham
London
N17 8DX

Helpline tel: 020 8801 7432
Admin tel: 020 8801 7432
Admin fax: 020 8885 3035
E-mail: projects@kitandkids.org.uk

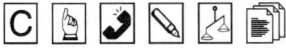

Description: A group of families facilitating the needs of their children, young and adult, who have a learning, physical and/or sensory disability. The aim is to integrate into society.

Index keyword: Disability: General Information

L

L'Arche

10 Briggate
Silsden
Keighley
West Yorkshire
BD20 9JT

Helpline tel: 01535 656186
Admin tel: 01535 656186
Admin fax: 01535 656426
Ie-mail: larche@ukonline.co.uk

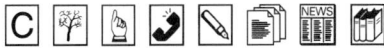

Description: L'Arche communities are places where people with and without learning disabilities live and work together in a simple way, to build community in an ecumenical Christian environment: places which offer a way of life that is not competitive, nor dependent on material success and intellectual achievement; places that heal rather than divide.

Index keyword: Mental Health/Illness

La Leche League

BM 3424
London
WCIN 3XX

Helpline tel: 020 7242 1278
Admin tel: 020 7242 1278
Opening times: 24 hours

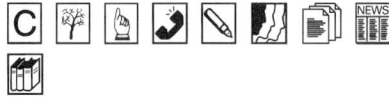

Description: Aims to encourage breast-feeding of infants.

Index keyword: Childcare

LADDER

P.O. Box 700
Wolverhampton
WV3 7YY

Helpline tel: 01902 336272
Admin tel: 01902 336232
Admin fax: 01902 336232

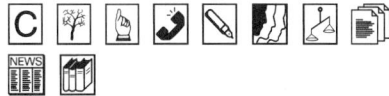

Description: Provides advice, information and support on all aspects of Attention Deficit/Hyperactivity Disorder.

Index keyword: Hyperactive Children

Lady Hoare Trust for Physically Disabled Children, The

1st Floor
89 Albert Embankment
London
SE1 7TP

Admin tel: 020 7820 9989
Admin fax: 020 7582 8251

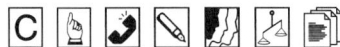

Description: The trust is committed to helping children, up to the age of 18, who have juvenile chronic arthritis or limb disabilities. A fieldwork team operates throughout the UK, offering practical advice. The trust also operates a small grants scheme.

Index keyword: Disability: Children

Larsen Syndrome Support Group

7 Littleworth Lane
Esher
Surrey
KT10 9PF

Helpline tel: 01372 467061

Description: The Larsen Syndrome Support Group is a self-help group, sharing experience and advice among families. It distributes the small amount of information available.

Index keyword: Larsen Syndrome

Latin American Women's Rights Service

Tindlemanor
52–54 Featherstone Street
London
EC1Y 8RT

Admin tel: 020 7336 0888
Admin fax: 020 7336 0555

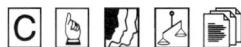

Description: The Service provides advice and support on immigration/welfare rights, health education, money and debt for Latin American women living in London. They also provide support for housebound women and a counselling service.

Index keyword: General Information

Learning Development Aids

Abbeygate House
East Road
Cambridge
CB1 1DB

Admin tel: 01223 357788
Admin fax: 01223 460557

Description: LDA develop materials for the mainstream primary curriculum. All publications are appropriate for children with specials needs.

Index keyword: Education

Leeds Antenatal Screening Service

26 Clarendon Road
Leeds
LS2 9NZ

Helpline tel: 0113 234 4013
Admin tel: 0113 234 4013
Admin fax: 0113 233 6774
Website: www.leeds.ac.uk/alss

Description: Leeds Antenatal Screening Service has been successfully providing private screening for Down's syndrome since 1991 and for cystic fibrosis since 1995. Women or healthcare professionals can contact their confidential helpline for further information, advice or to obtain sampling packs by post.

Index keyword: Pregnancy and Childbirth

Left Handed Company

PO Box 52
South DO
Manchester
M20 2PJ

Admin tel: 0161 445 0159
Admin fax: 0161 445 0159

Description: Supplies books and utensils for left-handers. Lectures/workshops available. Bibliographies/research papers. Mail order UK and worldwide.

Index keyword: Lefthanded

Legal Services Commission

85 Gray's Inn Road
London
WC1X 8TX

Admin tel: 020 7759 0000

Description: The Legal Aid Board is a non-departmental public body, set up under the Legal Aid Act 1988. It is responsible for ensuring the provision of legal advice and assistance to people in England and Wales of small or moderate means.

Index keyword: Advocacy

Leonard Cheshire Foundation

30 Millbank
London
SW1P 4QD

Admin tel: 020 7802 8200
Admin fax: 020 7802 8250

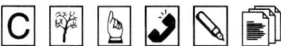

Description: Provides support for over 8,000 people with a wide range of disabilities and their carers, through its Care at Home, Residential and Nursing Services. In addition, it is involved in the development of independent and semi-

independent housing schemes. It also offers respite care, day services and rehabilitation, carries out assessment and provides counselling and training.

Index keyword: Disability: General Information

LEPRA (The British Leprosy Relief Association)

Fairfax House
Causton Road
Colchester
Essex
CO1 1PU

Helpline tel: **01206 562286**
Admin tel: 01206 562286
Admin fax: 01206 762151

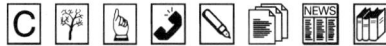

Description: LEPRA's aim is the eradication of leprosy. To that end the association raises funds in the UK to provide treatment for, and research into, the disease of leprosy.

Index keyword: Leprosy

Lesbian and Gay Bereavement Project

Vaughan M Williams Centre
Colindale Hospital
London
NW9 5HG

Helpline tel: **020 8455 8894**
Admin tel: 020 8200 0511
Admin fax: 020 8905 9250

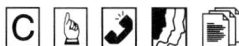

Description: Offers telephone and face-to-face counselling for lesbians and gay men bereaved by the loss of a same sex partner or otherwise affected by bereavement. Publishes a will form and is often able to find suitable clergy or secular officiants for funerals. Offers speakers and discussion leaders for any group concerned with death or dying.

Index keyword: Gays/Lesbians

Lesbian and Gay Christian Movement

Oxford House
Derbyshire Street
London
E2 6HG

Helpline tel: **020 7739 8134**
Admin tel: 020 7739 1249
Admin fax: 020 7739 1249
Opening times: Wed, Sun 10am–7pm

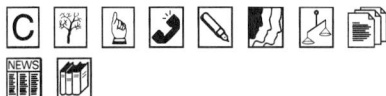

C

Description: Provides support to lesbian and gay Christians nationwide, through conferences, local groups, publications and membership services.

Index keyword: Gays/Lesbians

Lesbian and Gay Employment Rights

Unit 1g Leroy House
436 Essex Road
London
N1 3QP

Lesbian Helpline & Minicom: 020 7704 8066
Gay Helpline & Minicom: 020 7704 6066
Admin tel: 020 7704 2205
Admin fax: 020 7704 6067
Website: www.lager.dircon.co.uk
E-mail: lager@dircon.co.uk

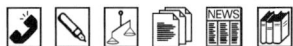

Description: Provides free and confidential advice to lesbians and gay men who are having problems at work.

The group provides training to individuals and organisations and also produces publications.

Index keyword: Gays/Lesbians

Lesbian Line

BM Box 1514
London
WC1N 3XX

Helpline tel: **020 7251 6911**
Admin tel: 020 7251 6692
Admin fax: 020 7608 0928

C

Description: Offers information, advice and support for all lesbians and training for volunteers.

Index keyword: Gays/Lesbians

Let's Face It

10 Wood End
Crowthorne
Berkshire
RG45 6OQ

Helpline tel: **01344 774405**
Admin tel: 01344 774405
Admin fax: 01344 762925

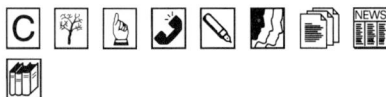

C

Description: This is a support network which links people with facial disfigurement, their families and friends, and professionals with resources for recovery.

Index keyword: Disfigurement

Leukaemia and Cancer Children's Fund

14 Featherhall Place
Edinburgh
EH12 7TN

Helpline tel: 0131 316 4149
Admin tel: 0131 316 4149
Admin fax: 0131 316 4060

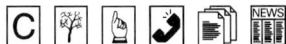

Description: Supports families throughout Scotland who have children suffering from leukaemia, cancer or similar blood-related disorders by offering holidays at their holiday home in Perthshire and limited financial assistance. Funds research at Yorkhill Hospital in Glasgow and provide an EPICS machine at the Royal Hospital for Sick Children in Edinburgh.

Index keyword: Cancer

Leukaemia Care Society, The

14 Kingfisher Court
Venny Bridge
Pinhoe
Exeter
Ex4 8JN

Admin tel: 01392 464848
Admin fax: 01905 330090

Index keyword: Leukaemia

Leukaemia Research Fund

43 Great Ormond Street
London
WC1N 3JJ

Helpline tel: 020 7405 0101
Admin tel: 020 7405 0101
Admin fax: 020 7242 1488
Website: www.leukaemia-research.org.uk
E-mail: info@leukaemia-research.org.uk

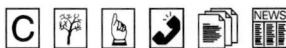

Description: The LRF is committed to preventing, improving diagnosis and curing all forms of Leukaemia, Myeloma, the Lymphomas and Hodgkin's Disease and related blood disorders such as Aplastic Anaemia and Myelodysplasma. It funds a national research programme, trains specialist doctors and provides comprehensive patient information. It depends entirely on voluntary donations.

Index keyword: Leukaemia

Life

Life House
1a Newbold Terrace
Leamington Spa
Warwickshire
CV32 4EA

Helpline tel: 01926 311511
Admin tel: 01926 421587
Admin fax: 01926 336497
Website: www.lifeuk.org
E-mail: info@lifeuk.org
Opening times: 9am–9pm

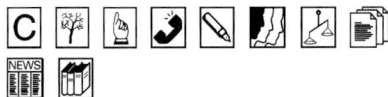

Description: Provides pro-life help and support to anyone with problem pregnancies or suffering after abortion. Also advises on accommodation for homeless mothers and gives talks in schools.

Index keyword: Abortion

Life Pregnancy Care Centre

83 Margaret Street
London
W1N 7HB

Helpline tel: 01926 311511
Admin tel: 020 7436 0777

C [icons]

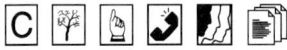

Description: Offers counselling for women facing pregnancy; provides free tests and free counselling: post-abortion counselling.

Index keyword: Pregnancy and Childbirth

Limbless Association

31 The Mall
Ealing
London
W5 2PX

Admin tel: 020 8579 1758

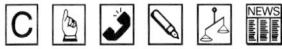

C [icons] NEWS

Description: Provides an information and advisory service for people of all ages who have been born without upper or lower limbs or have had amputations. Promotes rehabilitation through its home/hospital visiting service. Makes representation on policy matters to government departments, local authorities and health authorities.

Index keyword: Amputees

Link Centre for Deafened People

19 Hartfield Road
Eastbourne
BN21 2AR

Helpline tel: **01323 638230**
Admin tel: 01323 638230
Admin fax: 01323 642968
E-mail: linkcntr@dircon.co.uk

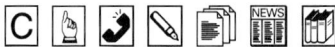

C [icons] NEWS

Description: Provides week-long residential rehabilitation courses for adults with severe or total hearing loss, together with their family or close friend. Aims to improve communication, personal adjustment and confidence.

Index keyword: Hearing Problems/ Deafness

Lissencephaly Contact Group

12 Didsbury Park
Didsbury
Manchester
M20 5LJ

Helpline tel: **0125 273 5470**

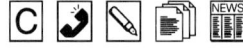

C [icons] NEWS

Description: Makes contacts among families with a child affected by lissencephaly; also provides information

Index keyword: Childcare

Listening Books

12 Lant Street
London
SE1 1QH

Admin tel: 020 7407 9417
Admin fax: 020 7403 1377
Website: www.listening-books.org.uk
E-mail: info@listening-book.org.uk

Living Paintings Trust, The

Queen Isabelle House
Kingsclere Park
Kingsclere
Newbury
Berkshire
RG20 4SW

Helpline tel: **01635 299771**
Admin tel: 01635 299771
Admin fax: 01635 299771
E-mail: lpt@livingpaintings.org

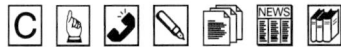

C [icons] NEWS

Description: Aims to enhance the lives of visually impaired people by providing access to the world of art through a specially designed audio-tactile system. Materials are available through a free national postal library service.

Index keyword: Blindness/Visual Handicap

Living Options

Kimbridge House
Kimbridge Road
East Wittering
Chichester
West Sussex
PO20 8PE

Admin tel: 01243 671865
Admin fax: 01243 671865

Description: Living Options provides small groups homes in the community for young people aged 18+ with disabilities.

London and Counties Society of Physiologists

330 Lytham Road
Blackpool
Lancashire
FY4 1AW

Admin tel: 01253 408443
Website: www.lcsb.uk.com
E-mail: lcsb@netcom.co.uk

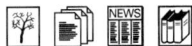

Description: The London and Counties Society of Physiologists, founded in 1919, is the country's oldest and largest organisation of private practitioners of remedial massage and manipulative therapy. It now represents around 2,000 practitioners and students of these professions.

Index keyword: General Information

London Bereavement Network

356 Holloway Road
London
N7 6PA

Helpline tel: **020 7700 8134**
Admin tel: 020 7700 8134
Admin fax: 020 7700 8146

Website: www.bereavement.org.uk
E-mail: info@bereavement.org.uk

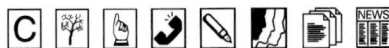

Index keyword: Bereavement

London Black Women's Health Action Project

82 Russia Lane
London
E2 9LU

Helpline tel: **020 8980 3503**
Admin tel: 020 8980 3503
Admin fax: 020 8980 6314

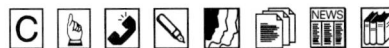

Description: Aims to promote the good and general well-being of black women in London; to campaign against the practice of female genital mutilation; to produce educational material for the community, voluntary and statutory sector; to develop a network of information and exchange with groups in the UK and internationally.

Index keyword: Women's Health

London Centre for Psychotherapy

19 Fitzjohns Avenue
London
NW3 5JY

Helpline tel: **020 7435 5512**
Admin tel: 020 7435 0873
Admin fax: 020 7435 1791

Description: Provides individual or group psychotherapy and counselling at moderate fees. Self-referral or referrals made by doctors, social agencies and other contacts are taken.

Index keyword: Psychotherapy

London Chinese Health Resource Centre

29–30 Soho Square
London
SW1V 5DH
Admin tel: 020 7287 0904
Admin fax: 020 7534 6545

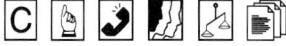

[icons]

Description: The Centre has a Sunday drop-in surgery where a bi-lingual (Chinese/English) doctor is on duty to provide health advice.

Index keyword: General Health

London Hazards Centre

Hampstead Old Town Hall
213 Haverstock Hill
London
NW3 4QP

Admin tel: 020 7794 5999
Admin fax: 020 7794 4702
Website: www.lhc.org.uk
E-mail: mail@lhc.org.uk

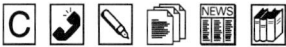

[icons]

Description: Provides advice, information and resources on health and safety at work and in the community in Greater London. Also carries out training, inspections and research.

Index keyword: General Information

London Lesbian and Gay Switchboard

P.O. Box 7324
London
N1 9QS

Helpline tel: 020 7837 7324
Admin tel: 020 7837 6768
Admin fax: 020 7837 7300

Website: www.llgs.org.uk
E-mail: admin@llgs.org.uk
Opening times: 24 hours

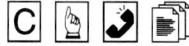

[icons]

Description: 24 hour helpline offering advice, support and information to lesbians and gay men and their families and friends. Minicom available.

Index keyword: Gays/Lesbians

London Lighthouse

111–117 Lancaster Road
London
W11 1QT

Admin tel: 020 7792 1200
Admin fax: 020 7229 1258

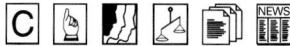

[icons]

Description: This is a residential and support centre for people affected by HIV and AIDS. Drop-in centre and cafe; community services; complementary therapies; creative therapies; day care; residential care: 23 beds offering respite, convalescent and terminal care; education, training and consultancy.

Index keyword: AIDS and HIV

London Rape Crisis Centre

PO Box 69
London
WC1X 9NJ

Helpline tel: 020 7837 1600
Admin tel: 020 7916 5466
Admin fax: 020 7916 5519
Opening times: Mon-Fri 6pm–10pm, Wed 10am–10pm.

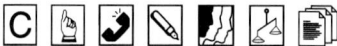

[icons]

Description: Counsels women and girls

THE HEALTH ADDRESS BOOK 2000–2001: A Directory of Health Support Groups

who have been raped/sexually assaulted, no matter how long ago. Advises on medical/legal matters and provides information and training on sexual violence issues. A limited advocacy service is provided.

Index keyword: Rape/Battered Women

Lupus UK

St James House
Eastern Road
Romford
Essex
RM1 3NH

Admin tel: 01708 731251
Admin fax: 01708 731252
E-mail:
headoffice@lupus-uk.freeserve.co.uk

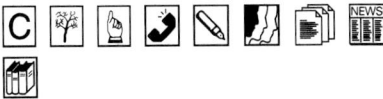

Description: Aims to educate the medical profession and the public about systemic lupus erythematosus and to raise funds for research and welfare and to support those diagnosed.

Index keyword: Lupus Erythematosus

Lymphoedema Support Network

St Luke's Crypt
Sydney Street
London
SW3 6NH

Helpline tel: **020 8748 2403;
020 8647 6456: 020 8650 2154**
Admin tel: 020 7351 4480
Admin fax: 020 7351 4480

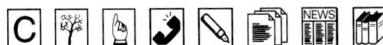

Description: Provides advice and support for sufferers of Lymphoedema.

Index keyword: Lymphoedema

M

Macfarlane Trust, The

Alliance House
12 Caxton Street
London
SW1H 0QS

Helpline tel: **020 7233 0342**
Admin tel: 020 7233 0057
Admin fax: 020 7233 0839

Description: Offers support to people with haemophilia who were infected with HIV from contaminated blood products in the UK.

Index keyword: AIDS and HIV

Make-A-Wish Foundation UK

Make-a-Wish House
Minster Court
Duscum Way
Camberley
GU15 3YY

Admin tel: 01276 24127
Admin fax: 01276 683727
Website: www.make-a-wish.org.uk

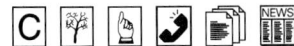

Description: Grants the favourite wishes of children suffering from life-threatening illnesses.

Index keyword: Childcare

Making Space

46 Allen Street
Warrington
WA2 7JB

Admin tel: 01925 571680
Admin fax: 01925 231402
E-mail: making.space@btconnect.com

Description: Helps schizophrenia sufferers in the north of England. Promotes practical help for schizophrenia and other mental illness sufferers and their families, with the provision of housing, supported residential facilities day centres and employment schemes. Family support workers available locally.

Index keyword: Schizophrenia

Male Advice Line and Enquiries (MALE)

PO Box 402
Sutton
Surrey
SM1 3TG

Helpline tel: 020 8644 9914
Admin tel: 020 8644 9914
Admin fax: 020 8543 8791
Opening times: Mon–Wed 9am–12am

Description: MALE offers help for male victims of domestic abuse and elder abuse; help for female perpetrators (relationships); and information/referral for male perpetrators.

Index keyword: Men's Health

Manic Depression Fellowship

Castle Works
21 St Georges Road
London
SE1 6ES

Admin tel: 020 7793 2600
Admin fax: 020 7793 2639
E-mail: mdf@mdf.org.uk

Description: Helps people with manic depression, their relatives, friends and others who care. Aims to educate the public and caring professions about manic depression and to encourage research for better methods of treatment. Produces a large range of publications.

Index keyword: Depression

Manic Depression Fellowship Scotland

19 Elmbank Street
Glasgow
G2 4PB

Helpline tel: 0141 331 0440
Admin tel: 0141 331 0440
Admin fax: 0141 331 0440

Description: The aims of MDF Scotland include helping people with manic depression, their friends, relatives and others who care; promoting, developing and co-ordinating a network of self-help groups throughout Scotland; maintaining a Scottish information and resource centre; improving knowledge and understanding of MD among professionals and the public.

Index keyword: Depression

Marfan Association UK

Rochester House
5 Aldershot Road
Fleet
Hampshire
GU13 9NG

Helpline tel: **01252 810472**
Admin tel: 01252 810472
Admin fax: 01252 810473
Website: www.thenet.co.uk/marfan

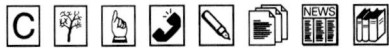

Description: Supports people with Marfan syndrome, provides educational material for both medical and lay sectors, and encourages research projects.

Index keyword: Marfan Syndrome

Margaret Hills Clinic, The

1 Oaks Precinct
Caesor Road
Kenilworth
Warwickshire
CV8 1DP

Helpline tel: **01926 854783**
Admin tel: 01926 854783
Admin fax: 01926 513133

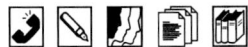

Description: Gives advice on ridding the body of excess acidity, which manifests itself as acid deposits, causing joint and muscle inflammation and pain. It can also appear as psoriasis, eczema, non-allergic asthma, bronchitis, migraine, headaches, kidney stones, gallstones, cystitis, sinusitis, catarrh, ulcers, colitis, diverticulitis etc.

Index keyword: General Information

Marie Curie Cancer Care

28 Belgrave Square
London
SW1X 8QG

Admin tel: 020 7235 3325
Admin fax: 020 7823 2380
Website: www.mariecurie.org.uk

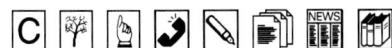

Description: Provides nursing and medical care for cancer patients in 11 hospice centres, and some 6,000 Marie Curie nurses who care for people in their own homes, throughout the day or night, free of charge.

Index keyword: Cancer

Marriage Care

Clitherow House
1 Blythe Mews
Blythe Road
London
W14 0NW

Admin tel: 020 7371 1341
Admin fax: 020 7371 4921
Website: www.mariagecare.org.uk
E-mail: mariagecare@btinternet.com

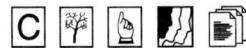

Description: Marriage Care is a national organisation which provides relationship counselling for individuals and couples; relationship education in schools. Marriage Care is a resource for parents, teachers and governors in planning and carrying out relationship education programmes; marriage preparation courses.

Index keyword: Marriage

Martin Street

Kids Clubs Network
Bellevue House
3 Muirfield Crescent
London
E14 9SZ

Helpline tel: **020 7512 2100**
Admin tel: 020 7512 2112
Admin fax: 020 7512 2010
Website: www.kidsclubs.co.uk
E-mail: information.office@kidsclubs.co.uk
Opening times: 9.00am–5.00pm

Index keyword: Childcare

Mary Martin School of Reflexology

72b Sharps Lane
Ruislip
Middlesex
HA4 7JQ

Helpline tel: **01895 635621**
Admin tel: 01895 635621

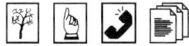

Description: The aim of the Mary Martin School of Reflexology is to produce competent and effective practitioners of reflexology to work with the general public in hospitals and the community; to convey the benefits of the therapy to the public through talks and leaflets. Support group for practitioners.

Index keyword: Complementary Medicine

Mary Seacole Nurses Association

52 Gledhow Park Avenue
Leeds
West Yorkshire
LS7 4JN

Helpline tel: **0113 262 3313; 0113 248 4727**
Admin tel: 0113 262 0282

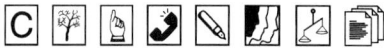

Description: Aims to raise awareness of health issues in black Afro-Caribbean elderly persons and to establish a non-profit-making nursing-home for frail black elders in the Chapeltown Leeds area.

Index keyword: Ethnic Minorities

Maternity Alliance, The

45 Beech Street
London
EC2P 2LX

Helpline tel: **020 7588 8582**
Admin tel: 020 7588 8583
Admin fax: 020 7588 8584
E-mail: info@maternityalliance.org.uk
Opening hours: vary – check recorded message on helpline.

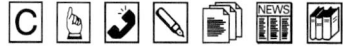

Description: Offers advice and information on maternity rights and benefits. If writing in, please enclose stamped self-addressed envelope for reply.

Index keyword: Pregnancy and Childbirth

Maternity and Health Links

The Old Co-op
38–42 Chelsea Road
Easton
Bristol
BS5 6AF

Helpline tel: **0117 955 8495**
Admin tel: 0117 955 8495
Admin fax: 0117 955 8495

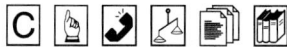

Description: Provides interpreting and advocacy for Asian families in their use of health services; information, advice, educational support on an individual and group basis for Asian families with health-related problems; an individual, home-based service for pregnant Asian women, focusing on English tuition and health education. Brings to the attention of health professionals and other statutory and voluntary bodies the needs of Asian communities.

Index keyword: Ethnic Minorities

Matthew Trust, The

PO Box 604
London
SW6 3AG

Admin tel: 020 7736 5976
Admin fax: 020 7731 6961
Website: www.matthew-trust.org
E-mail: matthewtrust@ukonline.co.uk

Description: Caring for the mentally distressed and victims of aggression.

Index keyword: Mental Health/Illness

MAVIS

DETR
'O' Wing
Macadam Avenue
Old Wokingham Road
Crowthorne
Berkshire
RG45 6XD

Admin tel: 01344 661000
Admin fax: 01344 661066
Website: www.mobility-unit.detr.gov.uk/mavis.htm
E-mail: mavis@detr.gov.uk

Description: The MAVIS is a mobility Centre offering driving ability assessments, advice and information on outside mobility. We can provide practical advice on driving, vehicle adaptation and suitable vehicle types for drivers and passengers.

Index keyword: Disability

ME Association

Stanhope House
High Street
Stanford-Le-Hope
Essex
SS17 0HA

Helpline tel: **01375 361013**
Admin tel: 01375 642466
Admin fax: 01375 360256

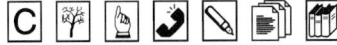

Description: Provides information and support to anyone affected by myalgic encephalomyelitis (ME). This includes literature, helplines, self-help groups, training and research.

Index keyword: ME (Myalgic Encephalomyelitis)

Mediation UK

Alexander House
Telephone Avenue
Bristol
BS1 4BS

Helpline tel: **0117 904 6661**
Admin tel: 0117 904 6661
Admin fax: 0117 904 3331

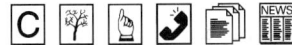

Description: Aims to make available conflict resolution skills, including mediation, to every citizen in pursuit of the promotion and protection of human rights. Exists to serve individuals, organisations and projects involved or interested in constructive approaches to handling conflict.

Index keyword: Mediation

Medic Alert Foundation

1 Bridge Wharf
156 Caledonian Road
London
N1 9UU

Helpline tel: **0800 581420**
Admin tel: 020 7833 3034
Admin fax: 020 7278 0647
Website: www.medicalert.co.uk
E-mail: info@medicalert.co.uk
Opening times: 9.00am–5.00pm

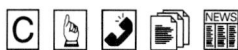

Description: Provides emergency identification, in the form of bracelets and necklets, for people with hidden medical conditions, such as diabetes, asthma, epilepsy and allergies.

Index keyword: General Information

Medical Action for Global Security (MEDACT)

601 Holloway Road
London
N19 4DJ

Admin tel: 020 7272 2020
Admin fax: 020 7281 5717
Website: www.medact.org
E-mail: info@medact.org

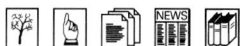

Description: MEDACT is a voluntary association of doctors and other health professionals in the UK working for the abolition of nuclear weapons, the promotion of peace and global security, the protection of the environment and preventive medicine on a global scale. It is the UK affiliate of International Physicians for the Prevention of Nuclear War, which won the Nobel Peace Prize in 1985.

Index keyword: General Information

Medical Advisory Services for Travellers Abroad (MASTA)

London School of Hygiene and Tropical Medicine
Keppel Street
London
WC1E 7HT

Helpline tel: **0891 224100**
Admin tel: 0906 822 4100

Description: MASTA's Travellers' Health Line (0891 224100) provides specific information on immunisations, malaria prophylaxis, the latest health news and any Foreign Office advice. The only charge is for the telephone call, which is a premium rate service.

Index keyword: Travel

Medical Council on Alcoholism, The

3 St Andrew's Place
Regents Park
London
NW1 4LB

Helpline tel: **020 7487 4445**
Admin tel: 020 7487 4445
Admin fax: 020 7935 4479

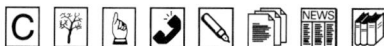

Description: Aims to educate the medical and allied professions about the effects of alcohol on health, for the benefit of their patients and themselves. Confidential organisation to help and assist with a drink/drug problem.

Index keyword: Alcohol Problems

Meet-A-Mum-Association

Waterside Centre
26 Avenue Road
South Norwood
London
SE25 4DX

Helpline: 020 8768 0123
Admin tel: 020 8771 5595
Admin fax: 020 8239 1153
Website: www.mama.org.uk
E-mail: Meet-A-Mum.Assoc@cablenet.co.uk
Opening times: 7.00pm–10.00pm

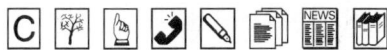

Description: Helps mothers who are isolated and lonely by putting them in touch with other mothers for friendship and support. Encourages the establishment of local groups. Offers information and one-to-one support to mothers suffering post-natal depression.

Index keyword: Pregnancy and Childbirth

Mens Health Matters

Petros Villas
69 Devizes Road
Salisbury
SP2 7LQ

Admin tel: 01722 339100
E-mail: iainsbury@petros-villas.u-net.com

Index keyword: Men's Health

Mencap (Royal Society for Mentally Handicapped Children and Adults)

117–123 Golden Lane
London
EC1Y ORT

Helpline tel: **020 7696 5593**
Admin tel: 020 7454 0454
Admin fax: 020 7668 3254
Website: www.mencap.org.uk
Opening times: 9.30am–5.30pm

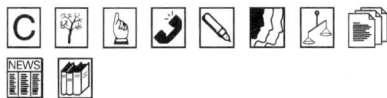

Description: MENCAP is exclusively concerned with people with learning disabilities and their families. The Society provides support and advice to individuals with learning disabilities and their families through its seven Divisional Officers, District Officers and a network of Local societies. MENCAP also runs residential services training and employment services and leisure services

through the National Federation of Gateways clubs and Mencap holidays. A monthly newspaper 'Viewpoint' is available through subscription.

Index keyword: Learning Disabilities

Mencap in Northern Ireland

Segal House
4 Annadell Avenue
Belfast
BT7 3JH

Helpline tel: **0845 7636227**
Admin tel: 028 9069 1351
Admin fax: 028 9064 0121
Website: www.mencap.org.uk
E-mail: mencap-ni@dnet.co.uk

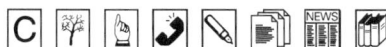

Description: Mencap is committed to campaigning for and providing high quality services and support. Its range of services include Segal House pre-school nursery, summer schemes, integrated play projects, parent to parent befriending schemes, family adviser information and advice services, Pathway employment placement schemes and residential services. It has a membership network of over 70 groups, with leisure opportunities being offered on a local level through its Gateway Clubs.

Index keyword: Learning Disabilities

Mencap's Holiday Service

Optimum House
Clippers Quay
Salford Quays
Manchester
M5 2XP

Helpline tel: **0161 888 1200**
Admin tel: 0161 888 1200
Admin fax: 0161 888 1214

C 👆 📞 ✏️ 🗐 📖

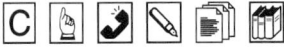

Description: Organises an annual programme of respite care breaks and holidays for unaccompanied children, young people and adults with a learning disability. These holidays include special care holidays for guests with profound intellectual and multiple disabilities; adventure, hotel and family-style holidays for more able guests; holidays abroad for adults.

Index keyword: Disability: Care Scheme/ Holidays

Meningitis Research Foundation

Midland Way
Thornbury
Bristol
BS35 2BS

Helpline tel: 080 8800 3344
Admin tel: 01454 281811
Admin fax: 01454 281094
Website: www.meningitis.org
E-mail: info@meningitis.org
Opening times: 24 hours; Office,
9.00am–5.15pm, Mon–Fri

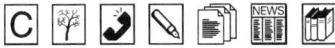

C 👆 📞 ✏️ 🗐 NEWS 📖

Description: Meningitis Research Foundation is fighting to prevent death and disability resulting from meningitis and associated infections by promoting awareness of the disease, and by working with affected families to raise funds for research into its prevention, detection and treatment.

Index keyword: Meningitis

Mental After Care Association (MACA)

25 Bedford Square
London
WC1B 3HW

Admin tel: 020 7436 6194
Admin fax: 020 7637 1980
Website: www.maca.org.uk
E-mail: maca-bs@maca.org.uk

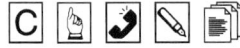

C 👆 📞 ✏️ 🗐

Description: MACA is a leading national charity offering a wide range of services for people with mental health needs and their carers including: advocacy, assertive outreach, community support, employment and day services, information and helplines, respite for carers, housing with support, schemes for people in contact with the criminal justice system, 24-hour access services.

Index keyword: Mental Health/Illness

Mental Health Act Commission

Maid Marion House
56 Hounds Gate
Nottinghom
NG1 6BG

Admin tel: 0115 943 7100
Admin fax: 0115 943 7101

🗐 📖

Description: The MHAC was set up to see that the Mental Health Act (1983) works well, and to look after the rights and concerns of all who may be held under the act. The commission is a group of about 90 people – doctors, nurses, social workers, psychologists, lawyers and others – with knowledge of the mental health service.

Index keyword: Mental Health/Illness

Mental Health Foundation Scotland

24 George Square
Glasgow
G2 1EG

Admin tel: 0141 572 0125
Admin fax: 0141 572 0246
Website: www.mentalhealth.org.uk
E-mail: mhf.scotland@btinternet.com

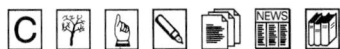

Description: Working on behalf of and with people of all ages with mental illness or learning disabilities. A grant-giving charity, also campaigning, educating and policy-influencing on relevant issues.

Index keyword: Mental Health/Illness

Mental Health Foundation, The

20–21 Cornwall Terrace
London
NW1 4QL

Admin tel: 020 7535 7400
Admin fax: 020 7535 7474

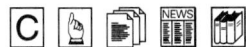

Description: As the UK's only charity concerned with both mental illness and learning disabilities. The foundation plays a vital role in pioneering new approaches to prevention, treatment and care. Its work includes allocating grants for research and community projects; contributing to public debate; educating and influencing policy-makers and healthcare professionals; and striving to reduce stigma and prejudice.

Index keyword: Mental Health/Illness

Mental Health Media

The Resource Centre
356 Holloway Road
London
N7 6PA

Admin tel: 020 7700 8171
Admin fax: 020 7686 0959
Website: www.mhmedia.com
E-mail: info@mhmedia.com

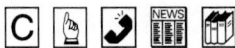

Description: Mental Health Media brings together the best from the media and the fields of mental health and learning difficulties in order to challenge discrimination and prejudice. Mental health media produces training and educational videos and resources, television, radio, CD ROMs, websites and other programmes which educate and inform. Mental health media offers training in media skills for users and professionals, provides media support for people who have experienced mental distress who want to be broadcast, and works to help journalists print and broadcast the voices of people who have experienced mental health problems.

Index keyword: Mental Health/Illness/Learning difficulties

Methodist Homes for the Aged

Epworth House
Stuart Street
Derby
DE1 2EQ

Admin tel: 01332 296200
Admin fax: 01332 296925
Website: www.methodisthomes.org.uk
E-mail: enquiries@methodisthomes.org.uk

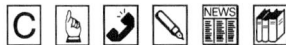

Description: Cares for older people in 41 residential homes, including a number of specialist homes for people with dementia. Befriending service, Live at Home, responds to the needs of older people in their own homes. Methodist Homes Housing Association manages 20 sheltered housing schemes for rent.

Index keyword: Elderly: Accommodation/Housing

Michael Palin Centre for Stammering Children

Finsbury Health Centre
Pine Street
London
EC1R 0LP

Helpline tel: **020 7530 4238**
Admin tel: 020 7530 4238
Admin fax: 020 7833 3842
E-mail: arsc@dial.pipex.com

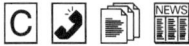

C 🤙 📑 📰

Description: Provides specialist assessment and advice for stammering children and their families from all parts of the UK. The centre supports local speech therapists in carrying out regular therapy and runs intensive courses in the Easter and summer holidays.

Index keyword: Speech Difficulties

Midlands Asthma and Allergy Research Association

12 Vernon Street
Derby
DE1 1FT

Helpline tel: **01332 362461**
Admin tel: 01332 362461
Admin fax: 01332 362462
Website: www.users.globalnet.co.uk/maara/index.htm
E-mail: jmcmaara@globalnet.co.uk
Opening times: 8.00am–5.00pm, Mon and Wed; 8.00am–3.00pm, Tues, Thurs and Fri

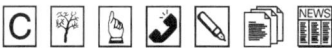

C 👁 ✋ 🤙 ✏ 📑 📰

Description: MAARA is a charity founded over 30 years ago to conduct and fund research into the cause and treatment of asthma and other allergies.

Index keyword: Asthma

Migraine Trust, The

45 Great Ormond Street
London
WC1N 3HZ

Helpline tel: **020 7831 4818**
Admin tel: 020 7831 4818
Admin fax: 020 7831 5174

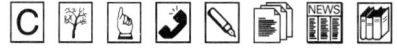

C 👁 ✋ 🤙 ✏ 📑 📰 📚

Description: Funds research into migraine, to improve diagnosis and treatment; holds international symposia; and provides help and information for sufferers.

Index keyword: Migraine

Mind (The Mental Health Charity)

15–19 Broadway
Stratford
London
E15 4BQ

Helpline tel: **020 8522 1728; 0845 7660163 (outside London)**
Admin fax: 020 8522 1725

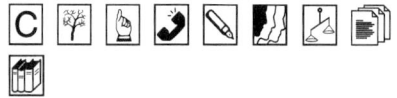

C 👁 ✋ 🤙 ✏ 🦶 📐 📑 📚

Description: Mind, the leading mental health charity in England and Wales, works for everyone experiencing mental distress; it campaigns for rights and promotes effective mental health services. Information and legal advice are offered, plus a legal network, publications, conferences and training.

Index keyword: Mental Health/Illness

Miscarriage Association, The

c/o Clayton Hospital
Northgate
Wakefield
West Yorkshire
WF1 3JS

Helpline tel: **01924 200799**
Admin tel: 01924 200795
Admin fax: 01924 298834
Website: www.thema.org.uk
Opening times: 9.00am–4.00pm, Mon–Fri

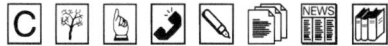

Description: This national charity
provides support and information for all
aspects of pregnancy loss. Gathers
information about causes and treatments
and promotes good practice in the way
pregnancy loss is managed in hospitals
and in the community. Has a network of
local contacts around the UK.

Index keyword: Pregnancy and Childbirth

Mobility Advice and Vehicle Information Service

TRL Crowthorne
Berkshire
RG45 6AU

Helpline tel: **01344 661000**
Admin tel: 01344 661000
Admin fax: 01344 661000

Description: The service was set up by the
Department of Transport to provide
practical advice on driving, car adaptations
and car choice for people with disabilities,
both as drivers and as passengers.

Index keyword: Disability: General
Information

Mobility Information Service

National Mobility Centre
Unit 2 Atcham Estate
Shrewsbury
SY4 4UG

Helpline tel: **01743 761889**
Admin tel: 01743 761889
Admin fax: 01743 761149

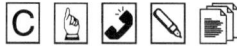

Description: Provides an information
service specialising in mobility problems;
driving assessment offered.

Index keyword: Disability: General
Information

Moor Green (Brain Injury Rehabilitation Unit)

Moseley Hall Hospital
Alcester Road
Moseley
Birmingham
B13 8JL

Helpline tel: **0121 442 4554**
Admin tel: 0121 442 4554
E-mail: mis@nmcuk.freeserve.co.uk

Description: Moor Green works to enable
people with brain injury to increase their
levels of independence in all areas of their
lives, thereby helping them to reintegrate
socially and enjoy an improved quality of life.

Index keyword: Neurological

Motability

Goodman House
Station Approach
Harlow
Essex
CM20 2ET

Helpline tel: **01279 635666**
Admin tel: 01279 635999
Admin fax: 01279 632000

Description: Motability exists to help get members on the road to freedom, by using their higher rate mobility component of Disability Living Allowance or War Pensioners' Mobility Supplement to buy or hire a car or wheelchair. Raises funds for adapted vehicles. Administers the government's mobility equipment fund and gives grants for specially adapted vehicles for people with the most severe disabilities.

Index keyword: Disability: Equipment

Mothers' Union, The

The Mary Sumner House
24 Tufton Street
London
SW1P 3RB

Admin tel: 020 7222 5533
Admin fax: 020 7222 1591

Description: The MU is specially concerned with all that strengthens and preserves marriage and Christian family life. Projects include work in prisons, 'away from it all' holidays and media awareness project. The Mothers' Union also does extensive work overseas.

Index keyword: General Information

Motor Neurone Disease Association

PO Box 246
Northampton
NN1 2PR

Helpline tel: **08457 626262**
Admin tel: 01604 250505
Admin fax: 01604 624726
Website: www.mndassociation.org
E-mail: enquiries@mndassociation.org
Opening times: 9.00am–7.00pm, Mon–Fri

Description: Supports peoples with MND and their families by providing advice and information, local support groups, a network of regional care advisers, an equipment loan service and limited financial assistance. Funds research into the cause of and a cure for MND.

Index keyword: Motor Neurone Diseases

Multiple Sclerosis Resource Centre (MSRC)

7 Peartree Business Centre
Peartree Road
Stanway
Colchester
Essex
CO3 5JN

Helpline tel: **0800 783 0518**
Admin tel: 01206 505444
Admin fax: 01206 505449
E-mail: themsrc@yahoo.com

Description: Informs and educates people with MS, families, carers and professionals about multiple sclerosis and its influences on daily life. Offers advice and support counselling as appropriate and refers to other agencies where necessary.

Index keyword: Multiple Sclerosis

Multiple Sclerosis Society in Scotland

The Rural Centre
Hallyards Road
Inglestone
EH28 8NZ

Helpline tel: **0808 800 8000**
Admin tel: 0131 472 4106
Admin fax: 0131 472 4099
E-mail: admin@mssociety-scotland.org.uk

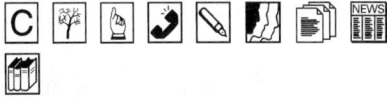

Description: Funds medical research into finding the cause of MS and a cure for it, and to improve the lot of people who have MS. The society's welfare role is exercised through its 45 branches throughout Scotland. It runs two holiday homes, and owns and lets out holiday caravans at several sites.

Index keyword: Multiple Sclerosis

Multiple Sclerosis Society, The

25 Effie Road
Fulham
London
SW6 1EE

Helpline tel: **0808 800 8000**
Admin tel: 020 7610 7171
Admin fax: 020 7736 9861
Website: www.mssociety.org.uk
E-mail: info@mssociety.org.uk
Opening times: Mon–Fri 9.00am–9.00pm

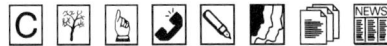

Description: Welfare and support service for people with MS and their families through a network of local branches. Holiday and short stay homes for members; raises funds for research.

Index keyword: Multiple Sclerosis

Muscular Dystrophy Group

7–11 Prescott Place
Clapham
London
SW4 6BS

Helpline tel: **020 7720 8055**
Admin tel: 020 7720 8055
Admin fax: 020 7498 0670
Website: www.muscular-dystrophy.org
E-mail: info@muscular-dystrophy.org

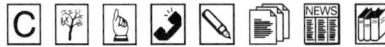

Description: This is the national charity funding research into treatments and cures for the muscular dystrophies and allied muscle-wasting conditions. Also supports adults and children affected by these conditions, with expert clinical care, counselling and grants towards equipment.

Index keyword: Muscular Dystrophy

Music for the Disabled

5 Guildown Road
Guildford
Surrey
GU2 5EW

Admin tel: 01483 567387
Admin fax: 01483 567387
E-mail: fred.weylec@ukgateway.net

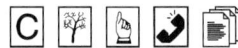

Description: Aims to provide live music entertainment/suffering from mental/physical disabilities in hospitals, schools and homes for the aged. Gives sessions of quiet live music for severely handicapped very young children.

Index keyword: Disability: General Information

Myasthenia Gravis Association

Keynes House
Chester Park
Alfreton Road
Derby
DE21 4AS

Admin tel: 01332 290219
Admin fax: 01332 293641
Website: www.crabby.demon.co.uk/mga/

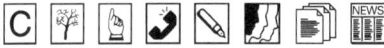

Description: Funds research to find improved treatments for the condition and an eventual cure. Also provides support and care for sufferers, their families and carers.

Index keyword: Myasthenia Gravis

Myelin Project, The

Douglas Cottage
2 Eshiels
Peebles
EH45 8NA

Helpline tel: 01721 720 546
Admin fax: 01721 723 474
Website:
www.myelinprobbritish.demon.co.uk
E-mail: hansec@myelinprobritish.co.uk

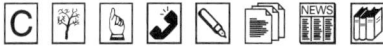

Description: Aims to accelerate research on the repair of the myelin sheath and restoration of lost functions in conditions like multiple sclerosis and leukodystrophies or neurodystrophies.

Index keyword: Multiple Sclerosis

N

NAPSAC

Department of Learning Difficulties
Floor e, South Block
University Hospital
Nottingham
NG7 2UH

Helpline tel: 0115 970 9987
Admin tel: 0115 970 9987
Admin fax: 0115 978 1598

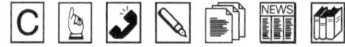

Description: Offers training on sexuality and personal relationships; protection from sexual abuse of both adults and children with learning disabilities; abusers with learning disabilities; policy guidelines for the prevention of sexual abuse of adults with learning disabilities.

Index keyword: Mental Health/Illness

Narcotics Anonymous

UK Service Office
202 City Road
London
EC1V 2PH

Helpline tel: 020 7730 0009
Admin tel: 020 7251 4007
Admin fax: 020 7251 4006
Opening times: 10am–10pm, 7 days a week

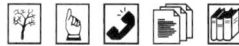

Description: Members encourage one another in recovery and in living as productive members of society; they carry the message of recovery to the still suffering addict.

Index keyword: Drug Addiction/Side Effects

National Abortion Campaign

The Print House
18 Ashwinn Street
London
E8 3DL

Admin tel: 020 7923 4976
Admin fax: 020 7923 4979

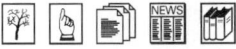

Description: Campaigns to ensure that all women have equal access to safe, free abortion on request; to raise awareness of the need for free, safe abortion; to increase awareness that a woman's right is crucial for women's autonomy and equality.

Index keyword: Abortion

National AIDS Helpline

Healthwise Helpline Ltd
1st Floor Caven Court
8 Matthew Street
Liverpool
L2 6RE

Helpline tel: **0800 567123**
Admin tel: 0151 227 4150
Admin fax: 0151 227 4019
E-mail: info@healthwise.org.uk
Opening times: 24 hours, 7 days

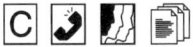

Description: Provides consistent and confidential information and advice on all aspects of HIV, including the routes of transmission of the virus, and on matters relating to HIV infection and associated illnesses, including AIDS, for anyone concerned about such matters throughout the UK. NAH also provides a UK-wide referral service to more specialist agencies. Also offers other information regarding sexually transmitted diseases.

Index keyword: AIDS and HIV

National Ankylosing Spondylitis Society

PO Box 179
Mayfield
East Sussex
TN20 6ZL

Admin tel: 01435 873527
Admin fax: 01435 873027

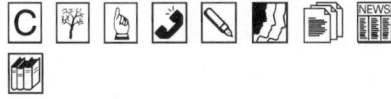

Description: Educates patients and provides physiotherapy in the evenings in 100 branches.

Index keyword: Ankylosing Spondylitis

National Association for Children of Alcoholics, The

PO Box 64
Fishponds
Bristol
BS16 2HH

Helpline tel: **0800 358 3466**
Admin tel: 0117 924 8005
Admin fax: 0117 942 2928

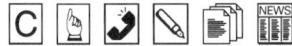

Description: Aims to raise the profile of children of alcoholics in the public consciousness; to reach professionals who deal with children of alcoholics in their everyday work; to offer advice, information and fellowship to children of alcoholics; to promote research into the phenomena of children of alcoholics.

Index keyword: Alcohol Problems

National Association for Colitis and Crohn's Disease

4 Beaumont House
Sutton Road
St. Albans
Hertfordshire
AL1 5HA

Helpline tel: **01727 844296**
Admin tel: 01727 862550
Admin fax: 01727 862550
Website: www.nacc.org.uk
E-mail: nacc@nacc.org.uk
Opening times: 24 hours answerphone

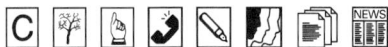

Description: Provides general information about inflammatory bowel diseases for sufferers, their relatives and friends. Encourages research into the treatment, management and causes of these diseases. Publishes booklets and quarterly newsletter for patients.

Index keyword: Crohn's Disease

National Association for Maternal and Child Welfare Limited

First Floor
40–42 Osnaburgh Street
London
NW1 3ND

Helpline tel: 020 8876 8070
(Dr Pryce-Jones)
Admin tel: 020 7383 4117
Admin fax: 020 7383 4115
Website: www.charitynet.org/-namcw

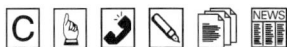

Description: Provides education and training in the broad field of child care and development. Holds annual study days on relevant topics.

Index keyword: Childcare

National Association for Patient Participation

The Chairperson
PO Box 999
Nuneaton
Warwickshire
CV11 6ZS

Helpline tel: 0151 630 5786
Answerphone: 0151 630 5786
Admin fax: 0151 630 5786
Website: www.napp.org.uk

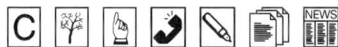

Description: The association helps doctors, practice managers and PCG's through a network of regional officers, to form and support patient participation groups in general practice; to enable the groups to air their views; to disseminate information and advice. The activities of these groups reflect the identified areas of need in the surgery. An affiliation process is available to newly formed and established groups.

Index keyword: Patients Rights

National Association for Premenstrual Syndrome (NAPS)

PO Box 72
Sevenoaks
Kent
TN13 1XQ

Helpline tel: 01732 760011
Admin tel: 01732 760011
Admin fax: 01732 760011
Website: ourworld.compuserve.com/homepages/nassupport
E-mail: nassupport@compuserve.com

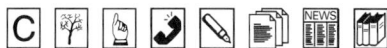

Description: The aim of NAPS is that any woman suffering from PMS should be able to get appropriate help quickly and easily for herself and those around her. NAPS runs training courses for prospective group leaders and/or telephone contacts. Organises seminars and lectures for health professionals.

Index keyword: Premenstrual Syndrome

National Association for Staff Support (NASS)

9 Caradon Close
Working
Surrey
GU21 3DU

Helpline tel: 01483 771599
Admin tel: 01483 771599
Admin fax: 01483 771599
Website: ourworld.compuserve.com/
homepages/nassupport
E-mail: nassupport@compuserve.com

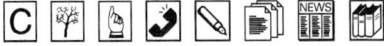

Index keyword: General Information

National Association for the Care and Resettlement of Offenders (NACRO)

169 Clapham Road
London
SW9 OPU

Helpline tel: 020 7582 6500
Admin tel: 020 7582 6500
Admin fax: 020 7735 4666
E-mail: communications@nacro.org.uk

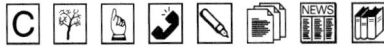

Description: NACRO works to prevent crime and promote the resettlement of offenders in the community by providing a wide range of practical services to offenders, to others at risk of offending, and to communities suffering from the effects of crime.

Index keyword: General Information

National Association for the Education of Sick Children (NAESC)

18 Victoria Park Square
London
E2 9PF

Admin tel: 020 8980 8523
Admin fax: 020 8890 3447
Website: www.sickchildren.org.uk
E-mail: naesc@ednsick.demon.co.uk

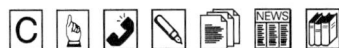

Description: Aims to ensure access and entitlement to good education for sick children; to encourage hospital trusts to adopt practices which contribute to effective education; to raise the profile of the subject; and to research the provision of education in hospital and at home.

Index keyword: Childcare

National Association for the Relief of Paget's Disease

323 Manchester Road
Walkden
Worsley
Manchester
M28 3HH

Admin tel: 0161 799 4646
Admin fax: 0161 799 6511
Website: www.paget.org.uk
E-mail: 106064,1032@compuserve.com

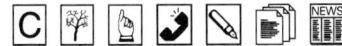

Description: Offers information and support to sufferers, directing them to appropriate treatment. Aims to raise awareness of the disease, and funds research into its causes and treatment.

Index keyword: Paget's Disease

National Association of Citizens Advice Bureaux

Middelton House
115–123 Pentonville Road
London
N1 9LZ

Admin tel: 020 7833 2181
Admin fax: 020 7833 4371
Website: www.nacab.org.uk

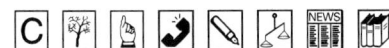

Description: Aims to ensure that individuals do not suffer through lack of knowledge of their rights and responsibilities, or of the services available to them; or through an inability to express their needs effectively and equally. The Association exercises a responsible influence on the development of social policies and services, both locally and nationally.

Index keyword: General Information

National Association of Councils for Voluntary Service

3rd floor Arundel Court
177 Arundel Street
Sheffield
S1 2NU

Admin tel: 0114 278 6636
Admin fax: 0114 278 7004
Website: www.nacvs.org.uk
E-mail: nacvs@nacvs.org.uk

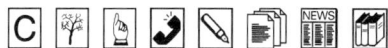

Description: Supports and develops local voluntary organisations through a network of Councils for Voluntary Service in England. Individual CVS hold details of voluntary organisations in their area. Contact NACVS for details of your local CVS.

Index keyword: Volunteers

National Association of Hospital and Community Friends

2nd Floor, Fairfax House
Causton Road
Colchester
Essex
CO1 1RJ

Admin tel: 01206 761 227
Admin fax: 01206 560 244
Website: www.info@hc-friends.org.uk
E-mail: info@hc-friends.org.uk

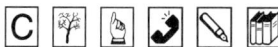

Description: The National Association of Hospital and Community Friends is the representative body for over 800 friends' groups working for the health, comfort and dignity of patients in hospital and the community. The Association is the support and advice centre for friends' groups, providing insurance, training, publications, grants, conferences and local support networks. Both written and telephone advice is available to members.

Index keyword: General Information

National Association of Laryngectomee Clubs

Ground Floor
6 Rickett Street
Fulham
London
SW6 1RU

Helpline tel: 020 7381 9993
Admin tel: 020 7381 9993
Admin fax: 020 7381 0025

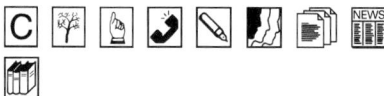

Description: The association promotes the welfare of laryngectomees and offers help and advice to all friends, family and professionals.

Index keyword: Disability: General Information

National Association of Toy and Leisure Libraries

68 Churchway
London
NW1 1LT

Helpline tel: 020 7387 9592
Admin tel: 020 7387 9592
Admin fax: 020 7383 2714

Website: www.charitynet.org/~NATLL
E-mail: admin@natl.ukf.net

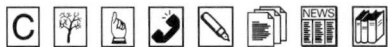

C 🌳 ✋ 📞 ✏️ 📑 📰 📖

Description: Toy Libraries lend good quality, carefully chosen toys to families with young children, including those with special needs. Also offers a befriending, supportive service to parents and carers. Leisure Libraries extend this concept to adults with special needs.

Index keyword: Childcare

National Association of Widows

48 Queens Road
Coventry
CV1 3EH

Helpline tel: **024 7663 4848**
Admin tel: 024 7663 4848

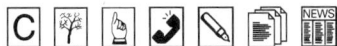

C 🌳 ✋ 📞 ✏️ 📑 📰

Description: Offers specific advice and information to all widows, their families and friends. Social support is available through branches and contract lists, including a list for younger widows.

Index keyword: Death and Bereavement

National Asthma Campaign

Providence House
Providence Place
London
N1 0NT

Helpline tel: 0845 7010203
Admin tel: 020 7226 2260
Admin fax: 020 7704 0740
Website: www.asthma.org.uk
Opening times: 9.00am–9.00pm, Mon–Fri

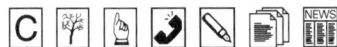

C 🌳 ✋ 📞 ✏️ 📑 📰

Description: The aim of the charity is to promote and fund research into asthma and related allergy, and to disseminate the results; to raise awareness of asthma and related allergy through media work campaigns, working with MPs and the government, and public education initiatives; to provide information, advice and support to people with asthma, their families and friends, health professionals, and the public.

Index keyword: Asthma

National Autistic Society, The

393 City Road
London
EC1V 1NG

Helpline tel: **020 7833 2299**
Admin tel: 020 7833 2299
Admin fax: 020 7833 9666

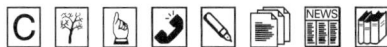

C 🌳 ✋ 📞 ✏️ 📑 📰 📖

Description: Offers information, advice and support to people who suffer from autism, and to their families and carers. Aims to improve awareness of the condition among key decision-makers, professionals and the general public. Provides training and promotes research.

Index keyword: Autism

National Benevolent Fund for the Aged

1 Leslie Grove Place
Croydon
CR0 6TJ

Admin tel: 0208 688 6655
Admin fax: 0208 688 1616
Website: www.nbfa.org.uk
E-mail: info@nbfa.org.uk

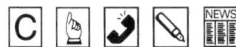

C ✋ 📞 ✏️ 📰

Description: Provides practical assistance to older people on low income, through the provision of TENS machines (for pain relief), emergency alarms (for independence), and holidays (for a change of scene and companionship).

Index keyword: Elderly: General Information

National Cancer Alliance

PO Box 579
Oxford
OX4 1LB

Admin tel: 01865 793566
Admin fax: 01865 251050

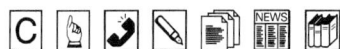

Description: The NCA is an alliance of patients and health professionals who are working towards improving the treatment and care of ALL cancer patients countrywide. They have established a track record of patient-centred research. They also provide information on cancer services and a directory of cancer specialists.

Index keyword: Cancer

National Childbirth Trust

Alexandra House
Oldham Terrace
Acton
London
W3 6NH

Helpline tel: 020 8992 8637
Admin tel: 020 8992 8637
Admin fax: 020 8992 5929
Website: www.nct-online.org

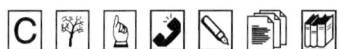

Description: Offers information and support in pregnancy, childbirth and early parenthood, and aims to enable every parent to make informed choices. Works towards ensuring that its services,

activities and membership are fully accessible to everyone.

Index keyword: Pregnancy and Childbirth

National Children's Bureau

8 Wakley Street
London
EC1V 7QE

Admin tel: 020 7843 6000
Admin fax: 020 7278 9512
Website: www.ncb.org.uk

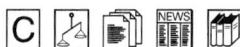

Description: A registered charity established in 1963, the National Children's Bureau seeks to increase awareness and understanding of the issues which affect children and young people. The charity aims to identify and promote the interests of all children and young people and to increase their status in a diverse society.

Index keyword: Childcare

National Consumer Council

20 Grosvenor Gardens
London
SW1W 0DH

Admin tel: 020 7730 3469
Admin fax: 020 7730 0191

Description: The National Consumer Council was set up by the government in 1975 to represent the interests of UK consumers of goods and services of all kinds, in both the public and private sectors. It is an independent body which campaigns, conducts research and supports other consumer organisations.

Index keyword: General Information

National Council for Hospice and Specialist Palliative Care Services

First Floor
34–44 Britannia Street
London
WC1X 9JG

Admin tel: 020 7520 8299
Admin fax: 020 7520 8298

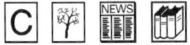

Description: Represents the views and interests of hospice organisations and palliative care services to government, the media and statutory and other agencies; and provides a forum for professionals working in palliative care teams to share knowledge, information and experience. Produces books for people working in hospices and palliative care services.

Index keyword: Pain

National Council for One Parent Families

255 Kentish Town Road
London
NW5 2LX

Admin tel: 08000 185026
Admin fax: 020 7482 4851
E-mail:
helpdesk@oneparentfamilies.org.uk

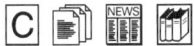

Description: Works to improve the economic, legal and social position of one-parent families. Offers an information service and training for professionals working with lone parents. Researches, lobbies and campaigns to improve the position of lone parents and their children. Lone Parents Into Employment projects are run at various locations, nation-wide.

Index keyword: Family Support and Welfare

National Council for Voluntary Organisations (NCVO)

Regent's Wharf
8 All Saints Street
London
N1 9RL

Helpline tel: **020 7713 6161 ext 2226**
Admin tel: 020 7713 6161
Admin fax: 020 7713 6300

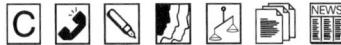

Description: NCVO champions the cause of the voluntary sector in England. Members range from large, household-name charities to small organisations, involved in all areas of voluntary and social action.

Index keyword: General Information

National Deaf Children's Society

15 Dufferin Street
London
EC1Y 8UR

Helpline tel: **0800 252380**
Admin tel: 020 7250 0123 engaged
Admin fax: 020 7251 5020

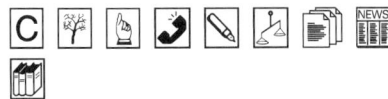

Description: This is an organisation of families, parents and carers which exists to enable deaf children to maximise their skills and abilities. Members include concerned professionals seeking to improve services for deaf children. A range of services is provided through national and regional staff.

Index keyword: Hearing Problems/ Deafness

National Deafblind League

100 Bridge Street
Peterborough
PE1 1DY

Admin tel: 01733 358100
Admin fax: 01733 358356

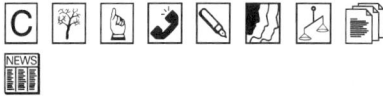

Description: Works to enable people with dual sensory impairment live full and active lives; to raise awareness of deafblindness in caring professions and the wider public; to ensure needs are met in health/community care planning. Visiting/assessing deafblind individuals, contributing to care plans. Social activities, rehabilitation services.

Index keyword: Hearing Problems/ Deafness

National Drugs Helpline

1st Floor
Cavern Court
8 Matthew Street
Liverpool
L2 6RE

Helpline tel: 0800 776600

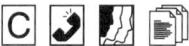

Description: The NDH is UK-wide and offers a comprehensive range of information advice and counselling about all aspects of drug misuse, including a leaflet and literature ordering service and referrals to local agencies. The service is available to anyone concerned about drug misuse, including drug users, their families, friends and carers. Calls are free and confidential.

Index keyword: Drug Addiction/Side Effects

National Eczema Society

163 Eversholt Street
London
NW1 1BU

Helpline tel: **020 7388 3444**
Admin tel: 020 7388 4097
Admin fax: 020 7388 5882
Website: www.eczema.org
E-mail: eczema@nes.comu-netcom

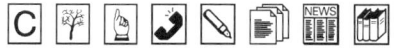

Description: Aims to improve the quality of life for people with eczema and their carers. Works to raise awareness of eczema and, through the Skin Care Campaign, works on behalf of people with skin conditions. Raises funds for research and organises professional education courses.

Index keyword: Skin Problems

National Endometriosis Society

Suite 50
Westminster Palace Gardens
1–7 Artillery Row
London
SW1P 1RL

Helpline tel: **020 7222 2776**
Admin tel: 020 7222 2781
Admin fax: 020 7222 2786
Website: www.endo.org.uk
E-mail: endoinfo@compuserve.com

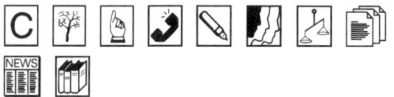

Description: Aims to enable sufferers and their partners and families to live with the condition. The service includes self-help groups, a helpline, specialist publications, workshops, advice and offers individual replies to medical questions.

Index keyword: Endometriosis

National Federation of 18 Plus Groups

Church Street Chambers
8–10 Church Street
Newent
Glos
GL18 1PP

Helpline tel: **01531 821210**
Admin tel: 01531 821210
Admin fax: 01531 821474

Description: The Federation, which is non-party in politics and non-sectarian in religion, seeks to assist people aged 18–36 to develop a personal philosophy and appreciate life, through the provision of opportunity for participation in cultural, social and recreational activities.

Index keyword: General Information

National Federation of Gateway Clubs

Mencap National Centre
123 Golden Lane
London
EC1Y 0RT

Admin tel: 020 7454 0454
Admin fax: 020 7608 3254

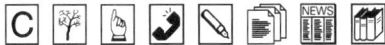

Description: Gateway aims to increase public awareness of the needs of people with learning disabilities and to ensure that they gain equal entitlement to community facilities.

Index keyword: Mental Health/Illness

National Federation of Retirement Pensions Associations

Thwaites House
Railway Road
Blackburn
BB1 5AY

Helpline tel: **01254 52606**
Admin tel: 01254 52606
Admin fax: 01254 52606

Description: Works to press for improvements to state pension and other state benefits for pensioners, by annual conferences and deputations to departments of state and all party group for pensioners at the House of Commons.

Index keyword: Elderly: General Information

National Federation of the Blind

The Old Surgery
125 Kirkgate
Wakefield
West Yorkshire
WF1 1JG

Admin tel: 01924 291313
Admin fax: 01924 200244
Website:
www.users.globalnet.co.uk/~NfBUK
E-mail: nfbuk@globalnet.co.uk

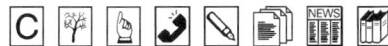

Description: Campaigns for integration of blind of partially sighted children in ordinary schools; for better employment for blind people; and for blindness allowance over the age of 16.

Index keyword: Blindness/Visual Handicap

National Foster Care Association

87 Blackfriars
London
SE1 8HA

Helpline tel: **020 7620 2100**
Admin tel: 020 7620 6400
Admin fax: 020 7357 6401

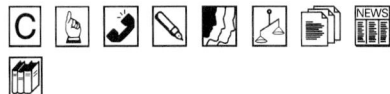

[C] [👍] [📞] [✏️] [🦶] [💡] [📑] [📰]
[📚]

Index keyword: Adoption and Fostering

National Heart Forum

Tavistock House South
Tavistock Square
London
WC1H 9LG

Admin tel: 020 7387 2799

[C] [📚]

Description: The National Heart Forum is the leading alliance of national agencies who work to reduce the UK's high rates of coronary heart disease.

Index keyword: Heart Problems

National Heart Research Fund

Concord House
Park Lane
Leeds
LS3 1EQ

Admin tel: 0113 234 7474
Admin fax: 0113 297 6208
Website: www.heartresearch.org.uk
E-mail: mail@heartresearch.org.uk

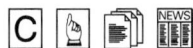

[C] [👍] [📑] [📰]

Description: Promotes medical research into heart disease and related disorders and into the prevention, treatment and cures of such complaints. Disseminates any useful results and provides practical help and rehabilitation for those with or vulnerable to heart disease or any related complaints.

Index keyword: Heart Problems

National Institute of Medical Herbalists

56 Longbrook Street
Exeter
EX4 6AH

Admin tel: 01392 426022
Admin fax: 01392 498963

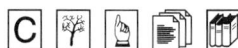

[C] [🌿] [👍] [📑] [📚]

Description: This is the UK's leading professional organisation of practitioners of herbal medicine (phytotherapy). Maintains high standards of practice and patient care, and works to promote the benefits of herbal medicine.

Index keyword: Complementary Medicine

National Kidney Federation

6 Stanley Street
Worksop
Nottinghamshire
S81 7HX

Helpline tel: **0845 6010209**
Admin tel: 01909 487795
Admin fax: 01909 481723
Website: www.kidney.org.uk
E-mail: mks@kidney.org.uk
Opening times: 9.00am–5.00pm, Mon–Fri

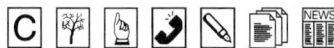

[C] [🌿] [👍] [📞] [✏️] [📑] [📰]

Description: Has 48 Member Associations and is the only national organisation in the UK that is run by kidney patients for the benefit of kidney patients. Represents patients' interest to government and the media; is active in campaigning to increase treatment facilities and encourages the public to look upon organ donation as the gift of life. Central office acts as an advice and information centre for patients and families, students, medical professions and general public.

Index keyword: Kidney Disease

National Kidney Research Fund and Kidney Foundation, The

Cirrus Court
Glebe Road
Huntingdon
Cambs
PE29 7EL

Helpline tel: **01480 398301**
Admin tel: 01480 356086
Admin fax: 01480 398303

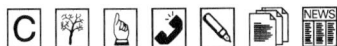

Description: Raises money for research and for patients' care and welfare.

Index keyword: Kidney Disease

National ME Centre

Disablement Services Centre
Harold Wood Hospital
Harold Wood
Romford
RM3 0BE

Admin tel: 01708 378050
Admin fax: 01708 378032
E-mail: nmecent@aol.com

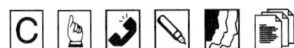

Description: The centre provides support for sufferers of ME in the management of their illness.

Index keyword: ME (Myalgic Encephalomyelitis)

National Meningitis Trust

Fern House
Bath Road
Stroud
Gloucestershire
GL5 3TJ

Helpline tel: **0845 600800**
Admin tel: 01453 768000
Admin fax: 01453 768001
Opening times: 24 hours
Website: www.meningitis-trust.org.uk
E-mail: support@meningitis-trust.org.uk

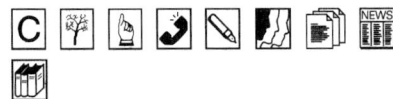

Description: Provides information and advice about meningitis to the general public and health professionals. Supports sufferers and their families with emotional, practical and financial support; and funds research into the disease.

Index keyword: Meningitis

National Music for the Blind

2 High Park Road
Southport
Merseyside
PR9 7QL

Helpline tel: **01704 28010**
Admin tel: 01704 28010

Description: Supplies a weekly music, news, comedy and plays service on a 90-

minute cassette to all blind and partially-sighted people.

Index keyword: Blindness/Visual Handicap

National Newpin

Sutherland House
35 Sutherland Square
London
SE17 3EE

Helpline tel: **020 7358 5900**
Admin tel: 020 7358 5900
Admin fax: 020 7701 2660
E-mail:
newpin@nationalnewpin.freeserve.co.uk

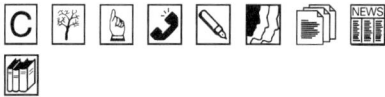

[C] [🌳] [✋] [📞] [✏️] [🦵] [📄] [NEWS]
[📖]

Description: National Newpin offers, through a network of local centres, a unique opportunity for parents and children to combat the emotional abuse which lies at the heart of child abuse. It works to achieve positive changes in their lives and relationships, based on the core values of respect, support, equality and empathy.

Index keyword: Childcare

National Organisation for Counselling Adoptees and Parents (NORCAP)

112 Church Road
Wheatley
Oxfordshire
OX33 1LU

Helpline tel: **01865 875000**
Admin tel: 01865 875000
Admin fax: 01865 875686

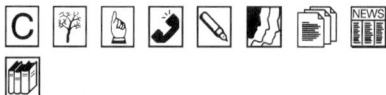

[C] [🌳] [✋] [📞] [✏️] [🦵] [📄] [NEWS]
[📖]

Description: Aims to provide support, guidance and sympathetic understanding to adult adoptees and their birth and adoptive parents. The organisation plays an intermediary role for people seeking renewed contact. Provides liaison with government, local authorities and adoption and fostering agencies. Also offers counselling services.

Index keyword: Adoption and Fostering

National Osteoporosis Society

PO Box 10
Radstock
Bath
BA3 3YB

Helpline tel: **01761 472721**
Admin tel: 01761 471771
Admin fax: 01761 471104
Website: www.nos.org.uk
E-mail: info@nos.org.uk
Opening hours: 10.00am–5.30pm, Mondays; 9.30am–5.30pm, Tues–Fri

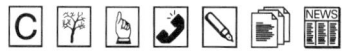

[C] [🌳] [✋] [📞] [✏️] [📄] [NEWS]

Description: This is the only charity working exclusively to improve the diagnosis, treatment and prevention of osteoporosis. Provides advice, information and support through a national medical helpline, a series of detailed information booklets and a network of local groups throughout the UK. It is an independent and unbiased organisation with its own specialist medical advisors.

Index keyword: Osteoporosis

National Playing Fields Association

25 Ovington Square
London
SW3 1LQ

Helpline tel: **020 7584 6445**
Admin tel: 020 7584 6445
Admin fax: 020 7581 2402
Website: www.npfa.co.uk
E-mail: npfa@npfa.co.uk

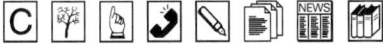

C ⟦icons⟧

Description: The National Playing Fields Association is the only national organisation which has specific responsibility for acquiring, protecting and improving playing fields, playgrounds and playspace where they are most needed and for those who need them most – in particular, children of all ages and people with disabilities.

Index keyword: General Information

National Radiological Protection Board

Chilton
Didcot
Oxon
OX11 0RQ

Helpline tel: **01235 822742; 01235 822744**
Admin fax: 01235 822746
Website: www.nrpb.org.uk
E-mail: information@nrpb.org.uk

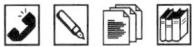

⟦icons⟧

Description: The National Radiological Protection Board (NRPB) is an independent statutory body, providing information and advice to persons, including government departments and the general public, on both ionising and non-ionising radiations. This covers x-rays, exposure to ultra-violet radiation and the health effects of electromagnetic radiation.

Index keyword: General Information

National Register of Hypnotherapists and Psychotherapists

12 Cross Street
Nelson
Lancashire
BB9 7EN

Helpline tel: **01282 716839**
Admin tel: 01282 699378
Admin fax: 01282 698633
Website: www.nrhp.co.uk
E-mail: nrhp@btconnect.com
Opening times: 9.00am–5.00pm, Weekdays

⟦icons⟧

Description: Provides referral service for members of the public seeking a qualified hypno-psychotherapist. Members are trained by the National College of Hypnosis & Psychotherapy and must abide by a code of ethics and carry appropriate insurance.

Index keyword: Psychotherapy

National Reye's Syndrome Foundation of the UK

15 Nicholas Gardens
Pyrford
Woking
Surrey
GU22 8SD

Helpline tel: **01932 346843**
Admin tel: 01932 346843
Admin fax: 01932 343920

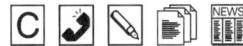

C ⟦icons⟧

Description: The charity was formed to provide funds for research into the cause, treatment, cure and prevention of Reye's syndrome and Reye-like illnesses; to inform both the public and medical communities; and to provide support for parents whose children have suffered from these diseases.

Index keyword: Reye's Syndrome

National Schizophrenia Fellowship (NSF)

Head Office
30 Tabernacle Street
London
EC2A 4DD

Helpline tel: **020 8974 6814**
(advice line open 10.00am–3.00pm
Weekdays)
Admin tel: 020 7330 9100
Admin fax: 020 7330 9102
Website: www.nsf.org.uk
E-mail: info@nsf.org.uk

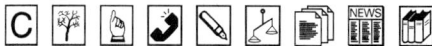

Description: The NSF is the largest
national voluntary organisation for
people with a severe mental illness, their
families and carers. It campaigns for
better services for the mentally ill and for
greater understanding of the problems
caused by severe mental illness,
particularly schizophrenia and related
conditions. NSF has approximately 6,900
members, over 170 carer and user self
help support groups around the UK.
Head Office is in London and there are a
number of core offices throughout
England, Wales and Northern Ireland.
NSF runs over 300 community care
projects across the UK ranging from
supported accommodation schemes to
employment training courses and day
care centres. It also carries out social
research; organises training courses/
conferences and provides free,
independent advice through its national
advice centre. NSF produces a range of
publications, which are either free or
available for a small cost, along with a
quarterly magazine 'Your Voice'.

Index keyword: Schizophrenia

National Schizophrenia Fellowship (Scotland)

Claremont House
130 East Claremont Street
Edinburgh
EH7 4LB

Helpline tel: **0131 557 8969**
Admin tel: 0131 557 8969
Admin fax: 0131 557 8968
Website: www.nsfscot.org.uk
E-mail: info@nsfscot.org.uk

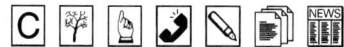

Description: NSF (Scotland) offers advice
and information to sufferers from mental
illness, their relatives and carers. Direct
services include day centres, employment
and training and carer support.

Index keyword: Schizophrenia

National Society for Epilepsy, The

Information Department
Chalfont St Peter
Gerrards Cross
Buckinghamshire
SL9 0RJ

Helpline tel: **01494 601400; 01494 873991**
Admin tel: 01494 601300; 01494 873991
Admin fax: 01494 871927
Opening times: 10am–4pm

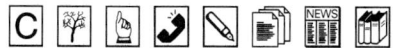

Description: The National Society for
Epilepsy provides assessment, treatment,
rehabilitation, long term care and respite
care for adults with epilepsy. The NSE is
at the forefront in epilepsy research and
has an information and education
department that runs a national helpline,
produces educational resources and runs
conferences and seminars. A community
network of support groups around the
country offers support and advice.

Index keyword: Epilepsy

National Society for Research into Allergy

PO Box 45
Hinckley
Leicestershire
LE10 1JY

Helpline tel: 01455 851546
Admin tel: 01455 851546
Admin fax: 01455 851546
E-mail: nsra.allergy@virgin.net

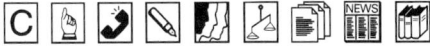

Description: Specialises in the detection of allergies/intolerances, candida, parasitic infection and has expert knowledge on tests/treatments and best doctors for all types of such problems. Also advises doctors, nurses and journalists.

Index keyword: Allergies

Nationwide Teetotallers Publicity Register

9 The Lodge
3 Blackwater Road
Eastbourne
East Sussex
EN21 4JF

Helpline tel: 01323 638234
Admin tel: 01323 638234

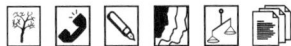

Description: Aims to introduce people who are seeking to follow an alcohol-free lifestyle to other teetotallers.

Index keyword: Alcohol Problems

Natural Death Centre

20 Heber Road
Cricklewood
London
NW2 6AA

Helpline tel: 020 8208 2853
Admin tel: 020 8208 2853
Admin fax: 020 8452 6434
E-mail: rhino@dialpipex.com

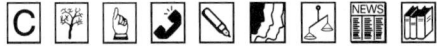

Description: This is a befriending network for people who are critically ill. Its services include volunteers visiting people at home to relieve carers; advice on inexpensive, green 'DIY' funerals; and a set of forms such as living will, advance funeral wishes and death plan.

Index keyword: Death and Bereavement

Natural Medicines Society

PO Box 232
East Molesey
Surrey
KT8 1YF

Admin tel: 020 8974 1166
Admin fax: 020 8974 1166
E-mail: NMS@charity-vfree.com

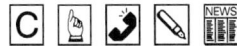

Description: The NMS represents the consumer voice for freedom of choice in medicine. Established in 1985, the Society aims to protect and develop the status of alternative and complementary medicine, working to ensure that the public has a genuine choice of treatments for their healthcare.

Index keyword: Complementary Medicine

NCH Action for Children

85 Highbury Park
London
N5 1UD

Admin tel: 020 7226 2033
Admin fax: 020 7226 2537

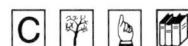

Description: NCH Action for Children is Britain's largest childcare charity – helping over 25,000 of the most vulnerable children and their families through 252 projects nationwide.

Index keyword: Children: General Information

Neurofibromatosis Association, The (NFA)

82 London Road
Kingston upon Thames
Surrey
KT2 6PX

Helpline tel: 020 8547 1636
Admin tel: 020 8547 1636
Admin fax: 020 8974 5601
Website: www.nfa.zetnet.co.uk
E-mail: nfa@zetnet.co.uk

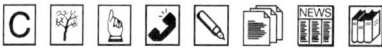

[C] [🌳] [☝] [📞] [✏] [📄] [NEWS] [📖]

Description: Provides a central point of contact for sufferers and information to professionals and the general public. Supports research into treatment and, ultimately, a cure for the condition. Aims to build a nation-wide network of neurofibromatosis support workers, who provide a supportive/counselling service to individuals and their families.

Index keyword: Neurofibromatosis

New Ways To Work

22 Northumberland Avenue
London
WC2N 5AP

Helpline tel: 020 7930 3355
Admin tel: 020 7930 0093
Admin fax: 020 7930 3366
Website: www.new-ways.co.uk
E-mail: nww@dircon.co.uk

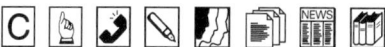

[C] [☝] [📞] [✏] [🦶] [📄] [NEWS] [📖]

Description: New Ways To Work campaigns and provides expertise on new and flexible ways of working that help people, organisations and society achieve a balance between work and the rest of life. Our aim is a society whose working culture gives real freedom of choice to people who cannot or do not wish to work traditional patterns. New Ways to Work is the acknowledged UK expert on flexible working arrangements, including part time work, job sharing, flexible working hours, term time working, career breaks, sabbaticals and working from home. New Ways to Work was founded in 1980 and achieved charitable status in 1983.

Main areas of work:
- Provision of information and advice on flexible working arrangements, via our Information and Advice Service and a range of expert publications.
- Running training sessions, conferences and workshops.
- Provision of commercial consultancy services to employers.
- Research and knowledge base development in all aspects of flexible working.
- Contributing to the development of public and government policy.

Index keyword: General Information

Newcastle Haemophilia Comprehensive Care Centre

Royal Victoria Infirmary
Newcastle upon Tyne
NE1 4LP

Helpline tel: 0191 232 5131
Admin tel: 0191 232 5131
Admin fax: 0191 230 0651

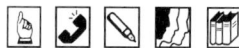

[☝] [📞] [✏] [🦶] [📖]

Description: The centre provides holistic care for people with bleeding disorders and their families.

Index keyword: Haemophilia

Newham Crossroads Care Attendant Scheme

Durning Hall
Earham Grove
Forest Gate
London
E7 9AB

Admin tel: 020 8555 8912
Admin fax: 020 8555 8912

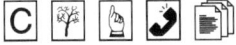

[C] [icon] [icon] [icon] [icon]

Description: Aims to provide carers in Newham with trained care support workers in order to give them a break from the stress and responsibility of looking after their disabled relatives/ friends.

Index keyword: Carers

NHS Confederation

Birmingham Research Park
Vincent Drive
Edgbaston
Birmingham
B15 2SQ

Admin tel: 0121 471 4444
Admin fax: 0121 414 1120

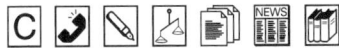

[C] [icon] [icon] [icon] [icon] [NEWS] [icon]

Description: The NHS Confederation represents the vast majority of NHS Trusts and Health Authorities, speaking for them uniquely on issues particular to each and in the context of the wide NHS.

Index keyword: General Health

NHS Direct

Victoria Health Centre
Glasshouse Street
Nottingham
NG1 3LW

Helpline tel: **0845 4647**
Admin tel: 0115 924 3328

Admin fax: 0115 941 3371
Website: www.nhsdirect.nhs.uk
Opening times: 24 hours

[icon] [icon]

Description: The service provides health information to the general public and to professionals in the following areas: illnesses and treatment, maintaining and improving health, NHS and related services, self-help groups, waiting times for treatment, how to complain about NHS services, and local NHS charter standards. The service is free to the user and information can be posted out.

Index keyword: General Health

NHS Health Information Service

College of Health
St Margarets House
21 Old Ford Road
London
E2 9PL

Helpline tel: **0800 665544**
Admin fax: 020 8983 1553
Opening times: Different for each area.

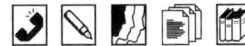

[icon] [icon] [icon] [icon] [icon]

Description: Provides information on medical conditions and treatments. Also provides advice on how and where to get treatment, hospital waiting times, medical procedures, self-help groups, complaints procedures and NHS services.

Index keyword: General Information

NHS Helpline

PO Box 5000
Glasgow
G12 9JQ

Helpline tel: **0800 224488**

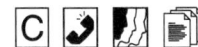

[C] [icon] [icon] [icon]

Description: The NHS Helpline Scotland is a free and confidential service providing a wide range of up-to-date health information, including: NHS services; patients' rights; waiting times; how and where to get treatment; free leaflets on medical conditions; local and national self-help groups and support organisations.

Index keyword: General Health

Nigel Clare Network Trust

Sonia Pemperton
85 Moorgate
London
EC2M 6SA

Helpline tel: **020 7256 8313**
Admin tel: 020 7256 8313
Admin fax: 020 7638 8648
Website: www.nigelclare.org
E-mail: postmaster@nigelclare.org

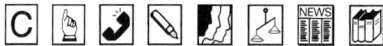

[C] [👐] [📞] [✏️] [👖] [⚖️] [NEWS] [📊]

Description: Gives practical advice to families caring for life limited children and youngsters by length, quality or by both, including income-earning help, support and advocacy publications, telephone help and advice.

Index keyword: Disability: Children

No Panic

93 Brandsfarm Way
Randlay
Telford
Shropshire
TF3 2JQ

Helpline tel: **01952 590545**
Admin tel: 01952 590005
Admin fax: 01952 270962
Opening times: 10.00am–10.00pm, every day of the year.

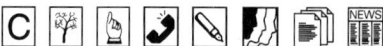

[C] [🌳] [👐] [📞] [✏️] [👖] [📄] [NEWS]

Description: Works for the relief and rehabilitation of people suffering from panic, phobias, obsessive compulsive disorder and related anxiety disorders; and offers support for their carers.

Index keyword: Phobias

Nordoff-Robbins Music Therapy Centre, The

2 Lissenden Gardens
London
NW5 1PP

Helpline tel: **020 7267 4496**
Admin tel: 020 7267 4496
Admin fax: 020 7267 4369
Website: www.nordoff-robbins.org.uk
E-mail: admin@nordoff-robbins.org.uk

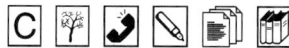

[C] [🌳] [📞] [✏️] [📄] [📊]

Description: In addition to being a clinic where children and adults can receive music therapy, the Nordoff-Robbins Music Therapy Centre offers a two year, full time training course in music therapy for professional musicians, leading to a Master of Music Therapy degree validated by the City University, London.

Index keyword: Complementary Medicine

North East Council on Addictions

Philipson House
5 Philipson Street
Newcastle-upon-Tyne
NE6 4EN

Admin tel: 0191 234 3486
Admin fax: 0191 263 9908

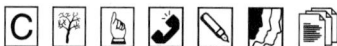

[C] [🌳] [👐] [📞] [✏️] [👖] [📄]

Description: Promotes the prevention, recognition and treatment of problems relating to the use of alcohol, drugs and related substances. Provides counselling, advice and support for users and non-users ie families and friends.

Index keyword: Alcohol Problems

Northern Ireland Chest, Heart and Stroke Association

21 Dublin Road
Belfast
BT2 7FJ

Helpline tel: **0345 697299**
Admin tel: 01232 320184
Admin fax: 01232 333487

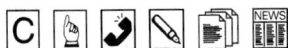

[C] [✋] [✆] [✎] [📄] [NEWS]

Description: Aims to prevent and alleviate chest, heart and stroke illnesses, through programmes of research, rehabilitation, welfare services and health promotion.

Index keyword: Heart Problems

Northern Ireland Community Addiction Service

40 Elmwood Avenue
Belfast
BT9 6AZ

Helpline tel: **02890 664434**
Admin tel: 02890 664434
Admin fax: 02890 664090
E-mail: nicas@dial.pipex.com

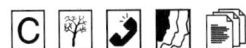

[C] [🌳] [✆] [🦶] [📄]

Description: This registered charity works at community level, providing a service for people who are abusing alcohol and drugs and people who are concerned about alcohol abuse. Aims to prevent problems in society and to provide a treatment service.

Index keyword: Alcohol Problems

Northern Ireland Polio Fellowship

198 Belvoir Drive
Belfast
BT8 4PJ

Helpline tel: **028 9064 3367**
Admin tel: 028 9064 3367
Opening times: 9am–10.30pm

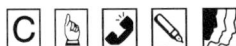

[C] [✋] [✆] [✎] [🦶]

Description: Helps members live as normal a life as possible. Housebound (and carless) members are taken shopping and on outings.

Index keyword: Polio

Norwood Jewish Adoption Society

Broadway House
80–82 The Broadway
Stanmore
Middlesex
HA7 4HB

Helpline tel: **020 8954 4555**
Admin tel: 020 8954 4555
Admin fax: 020 8420 6800
Website: www.nwrw.org
E-mail: norwoodravenswood@nwrw.org

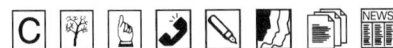

[C] [🌳] [✋] [✆] [✎] [🦶] [📄] [NEWS]

Description: Norwood Jewish Adoption Society is part of Norwood Ravenswood. The organisation is the largest Jewish child and family sevices charity in the UK. We are dedicated to supporting families and to promoting the best interests of children and young people. The adoption society offers both a domestic and inter-county adoption service.

Index keyword: Adoption

NSPCC

42 Curtain Road
London
EC2A 3NH

Helpline tel: **0808 800 5000**
Admin tel: 020 7825 2775
Admin fax: 020 7825 2763
Website: www.nspcc.org.uk
E-mail: infounit@nspcc.org.uk

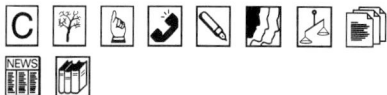

Description: Helps children and their
families through its child protection
teams, projects and national child
protection helpline. Also places strong
emphasis on the need to find out the
causes of child abuse and to work
towards its prevention.

Index keyword: Childcare

NSPKU

7 Lingey Lane
Wardley
Gateshead
Tyne and Wear
NE10 8BR

Admin tel: 08456 039136
E-mail: nspku@ukonline.co.uk
Opening times: 24 hour answerphone

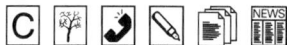

Description: Provides the opportunity for
people with phenylketonuria (PKU) and
their families to meet and share their
experiences. Disseminates information
and promotes the educational, medical
and social welfare of people with PKU.
Promotes and encourages regional
support groups around the country.

Index keyword: Phenylketonuria

Nursing Home Fees Agency (NHFA)

Old Bank House
95 London Road
Headington
Oxford
OX3 9AE

Helpline tel: **01865 750665**
Admin tel: 01865 750665
Admin fax: 01865 742157
Website: www.nhfa.co.uk
E-mail: admin-nhfa@msn.com

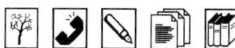

Description: Provides free specialist
financial/legal advice on entering nursing
homes and residential care. This includes
investment advice, local authority support
and duties, eligibility to DSS benefit. Aims
to enable elderly people to meet care costs
for life, whilst also preserving their capital
and, with that, their independence, dignity
and right of choice.

Index keyword: Elderly:
Accommodation/Housing

O

OASIS

Dan Y Graig
Balaclava Road
Glais
Swansea
SA7 9HJ

Helpline tel: **01792 844329**

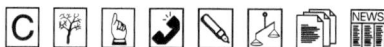

Description: OASIS helps people who
wish to adopt children from orphanages
in third world countries, and donates
money received to orphanages and
organisations caring for street children.

Index keyword: Adoption and Fostering

Oesophageal Patients Association

16 Whitefields Crescent
Solihull
West Midlands
B91 3NU

Helpline tel: **0121 704 9860**
Admin tel: 0121 704 9860
Admin fax: 0121 704 9860

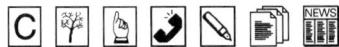

Description: The Association helps, encourages and supports oesophageal cancer patients by means of telephone advice from former patients, and information leaflets relevant to methods of treatment.

Index keyword: Cancer

Office for National Statistics

General Register Office
Adoptions Section
Trafalgar Road, Birkdale
Southport
PR8 2HH

Helpline tel: **0151 471 4831**
Admin tel: 0151 471 4831
Admin fax: 0151 471 4755
Website: www.ons.gov.uk
E-mail: adoptions@ons.gov.uk

Description: Provides adoption certificates, access to birth records for adopted people and an adoption contact register. Aims to link adopted people and their natural relatives.

Index keyword: Adoption and Fostering

One Parent Family Holidays

Kildonan Courtyard
Barrhill
Girvan
South Ayrshire
KA26 0PS

Helpline tel: **01465 821288**
Admin fax: 01465 821288

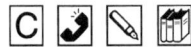

Description: One Parent Family Holidays was formed in 1975 by lone parents as a non-profit organisation. Their aim is to offer the chance of a continental holiday with others in a similar position.

Index keyword: Holidays

Open House Youth Counselling Service

Guildford YMCA Ltd
Bridge Street
Guildford
GU1 4SB

Helpline tel: **07932 047778**
Admin tel: 01483 565969
Admin fax: 01483 537161
E-mail: admin@guildford.ymca.org.uk
Opening times: 2.00pm–5.00pm, Mon, Tues, Thurs

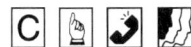

Description: Offers a free and confidential drop-in and booking counselling service to vulnerable young people and those who care for them. Offers individual counselling sessions on a one-off or long-term basis.

Index keyword: Counselling

Opportunities for People with Disabilities

123 Minories
London
EC3N 1NT

Admin tel: 020 7481 2727
Admin fax: 020 7481 9797
Website: www.opportunities.org.uk
E-mail: eopps.ho@care4free.net

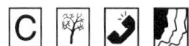

[C] [tree icon] [phone icon] [foot icon]

Description: Helps people with disabilities, through counselling, preparation and guidance, to secure employment matched to their talents and aspirations, by persuading employers to recognise ability and potential. Services are free to employers and disabled job-seekers from a network of regional centres.

Index keyword: Disability: Employment

Optical Consumer Complaints Service (OCCS)

PO Box 4685
London
SE1 6ZB

Helpline tel: **020 7261 1017**
Admin tel: 020 7261 1017
Admin fax: 020 7407 3991

[phone icon] [pencil icon] [book icon]

Description: OCCS is an independently managed service, the remit of which is basically the contractual element of a transaction with optometrists and/or corporate bodies. The function of the service is one of negotiation between practices and complainants where the patient has paid privately (not NHS).

Index keyword: Eye Care

Osteopathic Association Clinic

8–10 Boston Place
London
NW1 6QH

Helpline tel: **020 7262 1128**
Admin tel: 020 7262 1128
Admin fax: 020 7723 7492

[C] [phone icon] [book icon]

Description: The Clinic is dedicated to the furthering of osteopathic treatment, research and education.

Index keyword: Complementary Medicine

Osteopathic Centre for Children

109 Harley Street
London
W1G 6AN

Helpline tel: **020 7486 6160**
Admin fax: 020 7935 0019

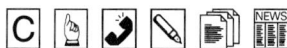

[C] [hand icon] [phone icon] [pencil icon] [document icon] [NEWS icon]

Description: Aims to treat children who cannot afford private treatment; educate osteopaths in paediatric osteopathy; instigate a programme of research into its effectiveness; raise public awareness that osteopathy is a suitable treatment for children.

Index keyword: Complementary Medicine

Osteoporosis 2000

47 Wilkinson Street
Sheffield
S10 2GB

Admin tel: 0114 272 2000
Admin fax: 0114 2634420

Index keyword: Osteoporosis

Osteoporosis Dorset

11 Shelley Road
Bournemouth
Dorset
BH1 4JQ

Admin tel: 01202 443064
Admin fax: 01202 443065
Website: www. dialspace.dial.pipex.com/osteo.dorset
E-mail: osteo.dorset@dial.pipex.com

Index keyword: Osteoporosis

OUTSIDERS

PO Box 28724
London
E18 1XW

Admin tel: 020 8220 5949
Admin fax: 020 8220 6963
E-mail: outsiders@beeb.net

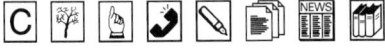

Description: Offers the physically and socially disabled the chance to meet new friends and gain the confidence to form new relationships. Friendly and informal events are organised in the London and Birmingham areas.

Index keyword: Disability: social

Overeaters Anonymous

PO Box 19
Stretford
Manchester
M32 9EB

Helpline tel: **0762 6984674**

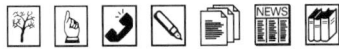

Description: Their primary purpose is to abstain from compulsive eating and to carry the message of recovery to those who still suffer. They take no position on outside issues and are not affiliated to any political movement, ideology or religious doctrine.

Index keyword: Eating Disorders

P

PACT

Sheffield Childrens Hospital
Western Bank
Sheffield
S10 2TH

Admin tel: 0114 2724570
E-mail: pact@sheffch-tr.trent.nhs.uk

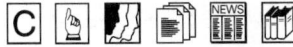

Description: PACT is the Parents Association of Children with Tumours and Leukaemia. Based at Sheffield Children's Hospital, it offers help to any family with a child referred to the oncology unit with cancer or leukaemia. It also funds vital research projects linked to Sheffield University. Also provides Home from Home accommodation and organises day trips and treats for the children.

Index keyword: Cancer

Paget Gorman Society, The

2 Downlands Bungalows
Downlands Lane
Smallfield
Surrey
RH6 9SD

Helpline tel: **01342 842308**
Admin fax: 01342 841540
Website: www.pgss.org
E-mail: PruP@compuserve.com

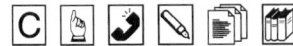

Description: Aims to help speech and language-impaired children to communicate and to develop an understanding of functional English through the use of Paget Gorman Signed Speech (PGSS), a system of manual signing which provides an accurate representation of spoken and written English.

Index keyword: Hearing Problems/ Deafness

Pain Relief Foundation

Pain Relief Foundation
Clinical Science's Centre
Univerisity Hospital
Aintree
Lower Lane
Liverpool
L9 7AL

Admin tel: 0151 523 1486
Admin fax: 0151 521 6155
Website: www.liv.ac.uk/pri
E-mail: pri@liv.ac.uk

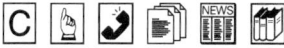

C 👍 ☎ 🗐 NEWS 📖

Description: Supports research (clinical) into chronic pain conditions; and postgraduate education (medical) in chronic pain management.

Index keyword: Pain

Pain Society

9 Bedford Square
London
WC1B 9RA

Admin tel: 020 7636 2750
Admin fax: 020 7323 2015
Website: www.staff.ncl.ac.uk/r.j.hayes/painsoc.html
E-mail: painsoc@compuserve.com

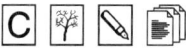

C 🌳 ✎ 🗐

Description: The Society was organised to relieve the suffering of pain by the promotion of education, research and training in the raising of standards in pain management.

Index keyword: Pain

Pancreatitis Supporters Network, The

15 Mayfield Court
59b Mayfield Road
Moseley
Birmingham
B13 9HS

Helpline tel: **0121 449 0667**
Admin tel: 0121 449 0667
Admin fax: 0121 449 0667

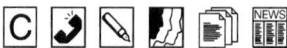

C ☎ ✎ 🦶 🗐 NEWS

Description: Gives advice, information and support to people with pancreatitis, their friends, family and workmates. Offers referral to pancreatitis specialists. Pain relief machines.

Index keyword: Pancreatitis

Parentline Plus

Highgate Studios
53–79 Highgate Road
Kentish Town
London
NW5 1TL

Parentline: 0808 800 2222
Admin tel: 020 7209 2460
Admin fax: 020 7209 2461
Website: www.parentlineplus.org.uk
E-mail: centraloffice@parentlineplus.org.uk
Opening hours: 9.00am–9.00pm, Mon–Fri; 9.30am–5.00pm, Sat; 10.00am–3.00pm, Sun

Description: Parentline is the confidential, freephone helpline run by Parentline Plus. It offers help and support to anyone in a parenting role. Staffed by parents trained in the issues callers raise.

Index keyword: General Information

Parent to Parent Information on Adoption Services (PPIAS)

Lower Boddington
Nr Daventry
Northamptonshire
NN11 6YB

Helpline tel: 01327 260295
Admin tel: 01327 260295
Admin fax: 01327 260295

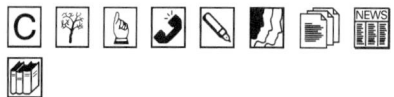

C 🌳 👍 ☎ ✎ 🦶 🗐 NEWS 📖

Description: Aims to assist people wishing to adopt, and also people who have adopted and need support; and to assist social workers in finding the right family for hard-to-place children.

Index keyword: Adoption and Fostering

Parentability (Disabled Parents Network)

PO Box 5876
Towcester
NN12 7ZN
Admin tel: 0800 018 4730
Admin fax: 020 7628 2833

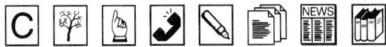

| C | 🌳 | 👆 | ☎ | ✏ | 📄 | 📰 | 📚 |

Description: Parentability is a National Childbirth Trust network of disabled parents. It supports them in pregnancy, childbirth and parenthood.

Index keyword: Pregnancy and Childbirth

Parenting Education and Support Forum

Unit 431
Highgate Studios
53–79 Highgate Road
London
NW5 1TL

Admin tel: 020 7843 6099
Admin fax: 020 7278 9512
E-mail: PESF@dial.pipex.com

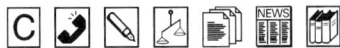

| C | ☎ | ✏ | 📐 | 📄 | 📰 | 📚 |

Description: Brings together those concerned or working with preparation, education and support for parents. Maintains a high profile for parenting education, supports and presses for effective policies and practices at local and national level, with the aim of serving the best interests of all children and their families.

Index keyword: Childcare

Parents At Work

45 Beech Street
Barbican
London
EC2Y 8AD

Right Advice Line: **020 7628 2128; 020 7628 3578 (answerphone)**
Admin tel: 020 7628 3565
Admin fax: 020 7628 3591
Opening times: 11.00am–2.00pm, Wed;
6.00pm–9.00pm, Thurs;
11.00am–2.00pm, Fri.

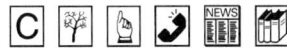

| C | 🌳 | 👆 | ☎ | 📰 | 📚 |

Description: Provides information on choosing childcare and obtaining a balance between work and home life, and also campaigns for better quality, affordable childcare for everyone. Works with employers to encourage family friendly practices in managers and policy makers.

Index keyword: Childcare

Parents for Children

41 Southgate Road
London
N1 3JP

Admin tel: 020 7359 7530
Admin fax: 020 7226 7840

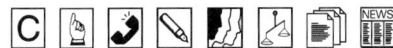

| C | 👆 | ☎ | ✏ | 🦶 | 📐 | 📄 | 📰 |
| 📚 |

Description: Parents for Children was founded in 1976 to find families for children considered children of exceptional needs. They now specialise in finding families for older children who have been abused, often sexually, are emotionally disturbed, sometimes mentally and physically disabled. They then provide a post-placement support service whenever the families feel the need.

Index keyword: Adoption and Fostering

Parents of Young Gamblers

14 Jasmin Croft
Kings Heath
Birmingham
B14 5AX

Helpline tel: **0121 443 2609**
Admin tel: 0121 443 2609
Admin fax: 0121 624 4626

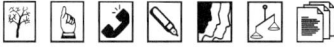

Description: Aims to persuade government in power to implement laws to stop children under 18 years having access to gambling activities, in particular fruit machines and lottery scratch cards.

Index keyword: Gambling

Parents' Friend

c/o Voluntary Action Leeds
34 Lupton Street
Leeds
LS10 5AX

Helpline tel: **01902 820497**
Admin fax: 0113 294 9677
Website: www.parentsfriend.demon.co.uk

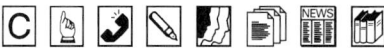

Description: Parents' Friend is a registered charity and is run by and for parents with lesbian, gay or bisexual offspring.

Index keyword: Gays/Lesbians

Parkinson's Disease Society

215 Vauxhall Bridge Road
London
SW1V 1EJ

Admin tel: 020 7931 8080
Admin fax: 020 7233 9908
E-mail: mailbox@pdsnk.demon.co.uk

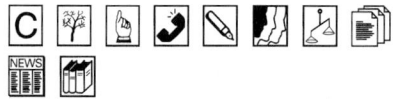

Description: Helps patients and their relatives with problems arising from the disease; collects and disseminates information; encourages and provides funds for research.

Index keyword: Parkinson's Disease

Partially Sighted Society

9 Plato Place
72–74 St Dionis Road
London
SW6 4TU

Admin tel: 020 7371 0289
Admin fax: 020 7371 0289

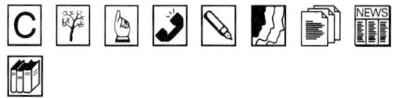

Description: Provides support, advice and information to visually impaired people and their families.

Index keyword: Blindness/Visual Handicap

Patients Association

PO Box 395
Harrow
Middlesex
HA1 3XJ

Helpline tel: **0845 6084455**
Admin tel: 020 7423 9111
Admin fax: 020 7423 9119
Website: www.patients-association.com
E-mail: mailbox@patients-association.com
Opening times: 10.00am–3.30pm

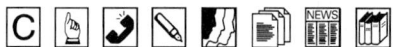

Description: Represent patients' interests to Government and professional bodies and all organisations involved in health matters. Offers support and advice to patients by telephone or correspondence. Produces a quarterly newsletter and a series of patient information leaflets.

Index keyword: Patients Rights

Pedestrians Association

31–33 Bondway
London
SW8 1SJ

Helpline tel: 020 7490 0750
Admin fax: 020 7820 8208
Website: www.pedestrians.org.uk
E-mail: info@pedestrians.org.uk

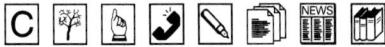

Description: Campaigns for the rights and safety of pedestrians, to improve the walking environment and to encourage more people to walk for short journeys. Promotes the 'walk to school' campaign and opposes bull bars on cars.

Index keyword: General Information

People First

Instrument House
207–215 Kings Cross Road
London
WC1X 9DB

Admin tel: 020 7713 6400
Admin fax: 020 7833 1880
E-mail: general@peoplefirst.k-web.co.uk

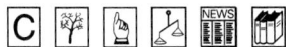

Description: Helps and supports people with learning difficulties to learn about speaking up for themselves on many different things in their lives. Runs training courses and produces accessible information on these issues. Campaigns for the rights of people with learning difficulties.

Index keyword: Education

Perthes Association

15 Recreation Road
Guildford
Surrey
GU1 1HE

Admin tel: 01483 34431
Admin fax: 01483 503213
Website: www.perthes.org.uk
E-mail: admin@perthes.org.uk

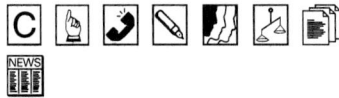

Description: Aims to help and advise families of children suffering from Perthes' Disease and Multiple Epiphyseal Dysplasia. Fund-raising for buggies, wheelchairs and other equipment, which are loaned free to members. Contributes to research programmes into the disease and other forms of osteochondritis.

Index keyword: Perthes Disease

PHAB England Limited

Sommit House
Wandle Road
Croydon
Surrey
CR0 1DF

Admin tel: 020 8667 9443
Admin fax: 020 8681 1399
Website: www.ukonline.co.uk/phab
E-mail: phab@ukonline.co.uk

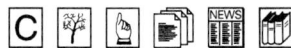

Description: Aims to promote and encourage people with or without physical disabilities to come together on equal terms and to achieve complete integration within the wider community.

Index keyword: Disability: Social

PHC

Thistledome Cottage
49 Main Street
Senstern, Grantham
Lincolnshire
NG33 5RT

Helpline tel: **01476 861379**
Admin tel: 01476 861379
Admin fax: 01476 861336

Description: Promotes the health and welfare of pet animals in the interests of both pets and people.

Index keyword: General Information

Philadelphia Association

17 Hampstead High Street
London
NW3 1QW

Admin tel: 020 7794 2652
Admin fax: 020 7794 2652
E-mail: paoffice@globalnet.co.uk

Description: This is an association of low cost, residential therapeutic communities in London. Psychoanalytic psychotherapy referral service (some low cost places). Training in psychoanalytic psychotherapy and phenomenology.

Index keyword: Psychotherapy

Phobics Society, The

4 Cheltenham Road
Chorlton-cum-Hardy
Manchester
M21 9QN

Helpline tel: **0161 881 1937**
Admin tel: 0161 881 1937

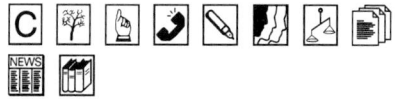

Description: The society offers help and guidance to people suffering from panic attacks, phobias and any obsessive compulsive disorders.

Index keyword: Phobias

Phoenix House

Central Office
47–49 Borough High Street
London
SE1 1NB

Admin tel: 020 7407 2789
Admin fax: 020 7407 6007
E-mail: phoenix.house@talk21.com

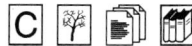

Description: Phoenix House is a national charity and special needs housing association, providing specialist care to substance misusers. Six residential centres, two residential family centres, three floating support schemes, three projects for people involved in the criminal justice system.

Index keyword: General Information

Pituitary Foundation, The

PO Box 1944
Bristol
BS99 2UB

Helpline tel: **01454 201612**
Admin tel: 0117 927 3355
Admin fax: 0117 927 3355
E-mail: helpline@ptpat.demon.co.uk

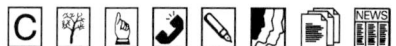

Description: Provides support and information to patients with rare pituitary conditions and their families or carers and increases public awareness of disorders. Builds networks of people who can offer mutual support.

Index keyword: General Information

Plain English Campaign

PO Box 3
New Mills
High Peak
SK22 4QP

Helpline tel: **01663 744409**
Admin tel: 01663 744409
Admin fax: 01663 747038
Website: www.plainenglish.co.uk
E-mail: info@plainenglish.co.uk

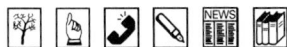

Description: Plain English Campaign is an independent organisation. It takes up the grievances of ordinary people who have been baffled by the bureaucratic language, small print and legalese of official information. The campaign is funded by its own commercial section which provides editing, writing, design and training services.

Index keyword: General Information

Playback Recording Service for the Blind

17 Gullane Street
Glasgow
G11 6AH

Admin tel: 0141 334 2983
Admin fax: 0141 334 2983
E-mail: playback@btinternet.com

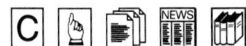

Description: Playback is a comprehensive recording service providing newspapers, magazines, reading service and tape library. The Playback Service will record anything requested for an individual or

organisation, if it is not available from another source and copyright clearance has been given.

Index keyword: Blindness/Visual Handicap

PMS Help

PO Box 83
Hereford
HR4 8YB
Admin tel: 01432 760993
Admin fax: 01432 760993

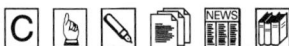

Description: Helps sufferers from premenstrual syndrome (PMS) and postnatal depression (PND) and their families, being aware that the families too experience the effects of these recurring hormonal diseases. Assists the medical profession in understanding PMS and PND.

Index keyword: Premenstrual Syndrome

Polyarteritis Contact List (Vasculitis Support Group)

15 Chepstow Grove
Birmingham
B45 8EG

Helpline tel: **0121 453 3349**
Admin tel: 0121 453 3349
E-mail: mg@gentle5.freeserve.co.uk

Description: Provides initial information for people with this rare illness. Updates and circulates annually a contact list of people with polyarteritis.

Index keyword: Polyarteritis

Porencephaly Contact Group

3 St Johns Hill
Ryde
Isle of Wight
PO33 1HN

Admin tel: 01983 563595

Description: The group places affected families in touch with each other.

Index keyword: Disability: General Information

Positive Partners/ Positively Children

Unit F7
Shakespeare Commercial Centre
245a Coldharbour Lane
London
SW9 8RR

Helpline tel: 020 7738 7333
Admin tel: 020 7738 7333
Admin fax: 020 7501 9382
E-mail:
clairebrighton@ppcs87.freeserve.co.uk

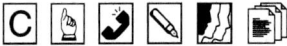

Description: Positive Partners, incorporating Positively Children, is an established charity providing practical and emotional support services to a wide range of people directly affected by HIV/AIDS.

Index keyword: AIDS and HIV

Positively Women

347–349 City Road
London
EC1V 1LR

Helpline tel: 020 7713 0222
Admin tel: 020 7713 0444
Admin fax: 020 7713 1020
E-mail: positivelywomen@dircon.org.uk

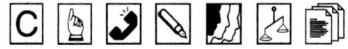

Description: Positively Women is the only registered charity offering peer support for women with HIV.

- Peer support and advocacy
- Creche facilities and therapeutic services for children affected by HIV
- Information and advice
- Training and volunteering opportunities
- Empowering women with HIV to make informed choices, ensuring the voice of HIV women is heard.

Index keyword: AIDS and HIV

Possum Controls Limited

8 Farmbrough Close
Stocklake
Aylesbury
Buckinghamshire
HP20 1DQ

Helpline tel: 01296 81591
Admin tel: 01296 81591
Admin fax: 01296 394349

Description: Possum provides a versatile modular range of environmental control equipment. Total solutions are ensured for people with a need to gain independence and easily control their security, communication, comfort and entertainment accessories.

Index keyword: Disability: Equipment

Post-Adoption Centre

5 Torriano Mews
London
NW5 2RZ

Helpline tel: 020 7485 2931
Admin tel: 020 7284 0555
Admin fax: 020 7482 2367
Website: www.postadoptioncentre.org.uk
E-mail: advice@postadoptioncentre.org.uk

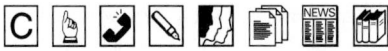

Description: Provides counselling and advice in order to meet the needs of both adults and children experiencing problems which arise in some way from adoption. Also provides workshops and professional training.

Index keyword: Adoption and Fostering

Prader-Willi Syndrome Association (UK)

2 Wheatsheaf Close
Horsell
Woking
Surrey
GU21 4BP

Helpline tel: **01483 724784**
Admin tel: 01483 724784
Admin fax: 01483 724784
Website: www.pwsa-uk.demon.co.uk

Description: The PWSA (UK) was founded in 1981 by a small group of parents, and now has over 500 family members and over 250 professional members. The Association aims to provide support and information to parents, carers, and people with PWS, and to promote knowledge and awareness of the syndrome amongst professionals and the public.

Index keyword: Prader-Willi Syndrome

Praxis Mental Health

29–31 Lisburn Road
Belfast
BT9 7AA

Admin tel: 01232 234555
Admin fax: 02890 245535

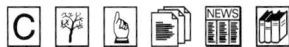

Description: Praxis is a charity which promotes mental health throughout Northern Ireland. It provides a range of services to people experiencing mental ill-health, including accommodation and support, volunteer befriending and 'Home Response', a domiciliary care service. The Praxis Research Department undertakes evaluations into the quality of the charity's work.

Index keyword: Mental Health/Illness

Pre-Eclampsia Society

12 Monksford Drive
Hullbridge
Hockley
Essex
SS5 6DQ

Description: Self-help and support group for sufferers of Pre-Eclampsia and Eclampsia.

Index keyword: Eclampsia

Pre-Eclampsia Society

Ty Iago Carmel
Caernarfon
Gwynedd

Helpline tel: **01286 880057**
Admin fax: 01286 880057

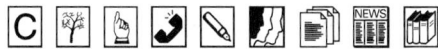

Description: This is a self-help and support group for sufferers of pre-eclampsia and their friends and families.

Index keyword: Pregnancy and Childbirth

Pre-School Learning Alliance

69 Kings Cross Road
London
WC1X 9LL

Admin tel: 020 7833 0991
Admin fax: 020 7837 4942
E-mail: pla@pre-school.org.uk

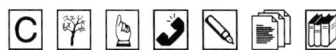

Description: Supports the education of children, primarily under school age, through parent-involving community groups. Supports such groups through training, publications, insurance and model constitution. Provides local advice and visits from field staff and volunteers at branch and county level; national office and eight regional centres.

Index keyword: Education

Pre-School Learning Alliance (South West Region)

54–56 Park Street
Bristol
BS1 5JN

Admin tel: 0117 907 7073
Admin fax: 0117 907 7074
E-mail: poole@pre-school.org.uk

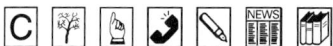

Description: The alliance, through its member groups, is the largest single provider of pre-school education and care in England. The alliance is a national educational charity committed to quality education and care for under-fives within a context of parental involvement and equal opportunities.

Index keyword: Education

Premenstrual Society

PO Box 429
Addlestone
Surrey
KT15 1DZ

Admin tel: 01932 872560 (Mon–Fri 11am–6pm)

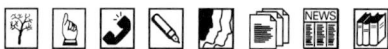

Description: Gives information and support to individual PMS sufferers and their families, provides educational courses on PMS, helps local support

groups etc and supports PMS research where possible. Newsletter available to members.

Index keyword: Premenstrual Syndrome

Prevention Of Professional Abuse Network (POPAN)

1 Wyvil Court
Wyvil Road
London
SW8 2TG

Helpline tel: **020 7622 6334**
Admin tel: 020 7622 6334
Admin fax: 020 7622 9788
E-mail: popan@easynet.co.uk

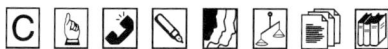

Description: POPAN provides information, advice, support and advocacy help for people who have been abused by health and social care professionals, promotes research and education of the public and professionals. POPAN aims to change existing policies and develop strategies to reduce, prevent and deal with abuse.

Index keyword: General Information

Primary Ciliary Dyskinesia (PCD) Family Support Group

67 Evendons Lane
Wokingham
Berkshire
RG41 4AD

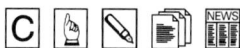

Description: Provides support to patients with PCD and parents of children with PCD. Aims to bring the disease to the attention of the medical profession and the public; to promote research; to aid diagnosis; and to improve treatment.

Index keyword: PCD

Prison Reform Trust

The Old Trading House
15 Northburgh Street
London
EC1V 0JR

Helpline tel: **020 7251 5070**
Admin tel: 020 7251 5070
Admin fax: 020 7251 5076
E-mail: prt@prisonreform.demon.co.uk

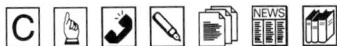

Description: The work of the prison reform trust is aimed at creating a just, humane and effective penal system. This is done by: inquiring into the workings of the system; informing prisoners, staff and the wider public; and influencing parliament, government and officials towards reform.

Index keyword: General Information

Professional Classes Aid Council

10 St Christopher's Place
London
W1M 6HY

Admin tel: 020 7935 0641

Description: Helps members of the various professions and their dependants in difficult circumstances.

Index keyword: General Information

Project for Advice, Counselling and Education (PACE)

34 Hartham Road
London
N7 9JL

Helpline tel: **020 7700 1323**
Admin tel: 020 7700 1323
Admin fax: 020 7609 4909
E-mail: pace@dircon.co.uk

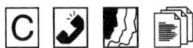

Description: This is a counselling organisation for lesbians and gay men. PACE also runs workshops and training courses for the statutory and voluntary sector. Now also operates Mental Health and HIV Advocacy service and Employment and retraining project.

Index keyword: Gays/Lesbians

Prostate Association

Stanley House
22 Paradise Street
Rugby
Warwickshire
CV21 3SZ

Helpline tel: **01788 643176**
Admin tel: 01788 330054
Admin fax: 01788 330056
Website: www.pha.u-net.com
E-mail: philip@pha.u-net.com

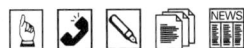

Description: Provides help, advice and information on prostate problems for sufferers, their families, and the media to educate the community at large over treatments and support.

Index keyword: Prostate

Psoriasis Association, The

Milton House
7 Milton Street
Northampton
NN2 7JG

Helpline tel: **01604 711129**
Admin tel: 01604 7111293
Admin fax: 01604 792894

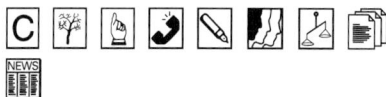

Description: Raises funds and promotes research into the basic causes of psoriasis and psoriatic arthritis, raising awareness of its problems and providing information on all aspects.

Index keyword: Skin Problems

Psoriatic Arthropathy Alliance

PO Box 111
St Albans
Hertfordshire
AL2 3JQ

Helpline tel: **01923 672837**
Admin tel: 01923 672837
Admin fax: 01923 672837
Opening times: 8pm–9.45pm

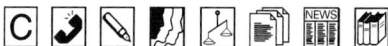

Description: The alliance is dedicated to raising awareness and helping people with psoriatic arthritis and its associated skin disorder, psoriasis.

Index keyword: Skin Problems

PSP Association, The

The Old Rectory
Wappenham
Nr Towcester
Northhamptonshire
NN12 8SQ

Helpline tel: **01604 860299**
Admin tel: 01327 860299/342
Admin fax: 01327 860923/1007
Website: www.PSPeur.org.uk
E-mail: psp.eur@virgin.net

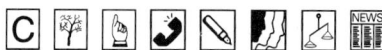

Description: Progressive supranuclear palsy is a progressive neurodegenerative disease affecting primarily vision, balance, swallowing and speech. A patient is usually confined to a wheelchair the last years of their life. Average life expectancy from onset is some seven years. The aims of the association are to promote research, engender awareness and provide information and support to carers and their families.

Index keyword: Neurological

Psychiatric Rehabilitation Association (PRA)

Bayford Mews
Bayford Street
London
E8 3SF

Helpline tel: **020 8985 3570**
Admin tel: 020 8985 3570
Admin fax: 020 8986 1334
Website: www.cityhack.dircon.co.uk
E-mail: ppra528898@aol.com

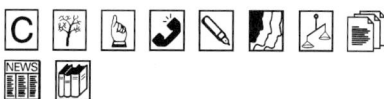

Description: Aims to stimulate patients towards greater initiative and social awareness; prepares and encourages patients to play an active part in their community. PRA is a partnership of patients, relatives, friends and professional workers. It has developed a wide range of community care facilities.

Index keyword: Mental Health/Illness

Psychotherapy Centre, The

67 Upper Berkeley Street
London
W1H 7DH

Helpline tel: **020 7723 6173**
Admin tel: 020 7723 6173
Website: www.the-psychotherapy-centre.freeserve.co.uk
E-mail: psychotherapy-centre@thewordsmith.freeserve.co.uk

Description: This is a long-established training, therapy, publishing, referral and research centre, with trained psychotherapists at the centre and elsewhere. Also gives information on training in psychotherapy.

Index keyword: Psychotherapy

Public Health Alliance, The

138 Digbeth
Birmingham
B5 6DR

Admin tel: 0121 643 7628
Admin fax: 0121 643 4541
E-mail: ukpha@ukonline.co.uk

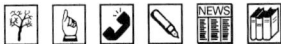

Description: Promotes and defends public health by means of conferences and seminars, publications, networking, lobbying and acting as an independent voice in advocating healthy public policy.

Index keyword: General Health

Purine Metabolic Patients Association (PUMPA)

71 Newcomen Street
London
SE1 1YT

Helpline tel: **020 7378 6079**
Website: www.pumpa.co.uk

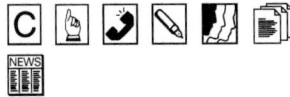

Description: Aims to offer help and advice to patients and families; also to educate the medical professionals to make proper diagnosis and give patients correct treatment.

Index keyword: General Information

Q

Queen Elizabeth's Foundation for Disabled People

Leatherhead
Surrey
KT22 0BN

Helpline tel: **01306 742282**
Admin tel: 01372 841100
Admin fax: 01372 844072

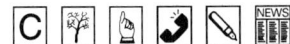

Description: A variety of services is offered to severely physically disabled adults. These include vocational training, information, day care, holidays, rehabilitation, employment, assessment, accommodation, mobility advice, respite care and further education.

Index keyword: Disability: General Information

Quit

Victory House
170 Tottenham Court Road
London
W1P 0HA

Helpline tel: **0800 002200**
Admin tel: 020 7388 5775
Admin fax: 020 7388 5995
Website: www.quit.org.uk
E-mail: quit-projects@clara.co.uk
Opening hours: 12.00pm–9.00pm, 7 days a week

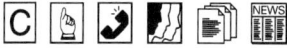

[C] [icons]

Description: QUIT is a national charity helping smokers to quit.

Index keyword: Smoking

R

Radionic

Baerlein House
Goose Green
Deddington, Banbury
Oxon
OX15 0SZ

Helpline tel: **01869 338852**
Admin tel: 01869 338852
Admin fax: 01869 338852
Opening times: 9am–1.30pm

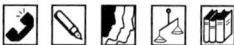

[icons]

Description: Radionics, a complementary therapy, is a method of healing at a distance through the medium of an instrument using the ESP faculty. Spring and autumn introductory weekends for prospective trainee practitioners. AGM and summer meeting in July.

Index keyword: General Information

Radiotherapy Action Group Expousre (RAGE)

24 Lockett Gardens
Trinity
Salford
Manchester
M3 6BJ

Helpline tel: **0161 839 2927**
Admin tel: 0161 839 2927
Admin fax: 0161 839 2927

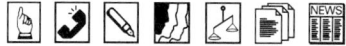

[icons]

Description: This is a free mutual support group for people who have a problem, physical or psychological, after radiotherapy treatment.

Index keyword: Cancer

Rainbow Trust

Rainbow House
47 Eastwick Drive
Great Bookham
Surrey
KT23 3PU

Helpline tel: **01372 453309**
Admin tel: 01372 363438
Admin fax: 01372 450699
E-mail: rainbowhouse@easynet.co.uk

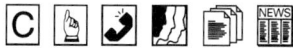

[C] [icons]

Description: Offers family-centred care for children with life-threatening or terminal illness.

Index keyword: Childcare

Rathbone CI

Head Office
Churchgate House
56 Oxford Street
Manchester
M1 6EU

Helpline tel: **0800 917 6790**
Admin tel: 0161 236 5358
Admin fax: 0161 238 6356
Website: www.rathbone-ci.co.uk
E-mail: advice@rathbone-ci.co.uk
Opening times: 10.00am–4.00pm, Mon–Fri

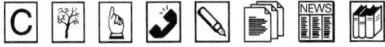

[C] [tree] [hand] [phone] [pen] [documents] [NEWS] [book]

Description: Aims to improve opportunities for people who have limited access to services, many of whom have learning difficulties and other special needs. Offers training, employment preparation and family support. National information line gives advice and information to parents, carers and professionals.

Index keyword: Mental Health/Illness

Ravenscourt (Alcohol and Drug Treatment Centre)

15 Ellasdale Road
Bognor Regis
West Sussex
PO21 2SG

Helpline tel: **01243 862157**
Admin tel: 01243 862157
Admin fax: 01243 867126
Website: www.ravenscourt.org

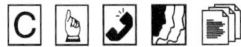

[C] [hand] [phone] [foot] [documents]

Description: This is a first stage treatment centre for addiction. It provides an abstinence-based programme of recovery within the setting of a therapeutic community for both men and women. It offers a safe environment in which personal recovery can take place. (No detox facilities).

Index keyword: Alcohol Problems

Raynaud's and Scleroderma Association

112 Crewe Road
Alsager
Cheshire
ST7 2JA

Helpline tel: **01270 872776**
Admin tel: 01270 872776
Admin fax: 01270 883556
Website: www.raynauds.demon.co.uk
E-mail:
webmaster@raynauds.demon.co.uk

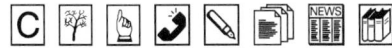

[C] [tree] [hand] [phone] [pen] [documents] [NEWS] [book]

Description: Offers advice and information to sufferers from Raynaud's scleroderma and associated conditions. Also funds research to find better treatments and gives practical support.

Index keyword: Raynaud's Disease

RCN Work Injured Nurses Group

20 Cavendish Square
London
W1M 0AB

Helpline tel: **020 8649 9536**
Admin tel: 01832 733177
Admin fax: 01832 733177

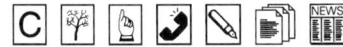

[C] [tree] [hand] [phone] [pen] [documents] [NEWS]

Description: Provides support and information to members of the Royal College of Nursing who have suffered injury or illness in the course of their work.

Index keyword: General Information

Reach

Reach Resource Centre
Wellington House
Wellington Road
Wokingham
Berkshire
RG40 2AG

Admin tel: 01734 891101
Admin fax: 01734 790989

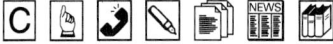

Description: Reach provides a resource and information centre for those who work with children whose disability, illness or learning problem affects their reading, language or communication. The centre contains printed books and books on sound tape and video, plus microelectronic equipment and software. The collections are reference only.

Index keyword: Disability: Children

REACH

89 Albert Embankment
London
SE1 7TP

Admin tel: 020 7582 6543
Admin fax: 020 7582 2423
Website: www.volwork.org.uk
E-mail: volwork@btinternet.com

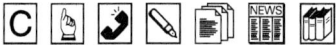

Description: REACH finds part-time expenses only jobs for professional people.

Index keyword: Volunteers

Reach (Association for Children with Hand or Arm Deficiency, The)

25 High Street
Wellingborough
Northamptonshire
NN8 4JZ

Admin tel: 01933 274126
Admin fax: 01933 274126
Website: www.reach.org.uk

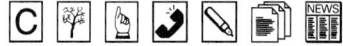

Description: The association provides contact and support for families with children who have any form of hand or arm deficiency.

Index keyword: Disability: Children

React

St Lukes House
270 Sandycombe Road
Kew
Richmond
Surrey
TW9 3NP

Helpline tel: **020 8940 2575**
Admin tel: 020 8940 2575
Admin fax: 020 8940 2050

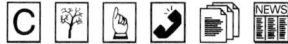

Description: React offers assistance and works to improve the quality of life for children with potentially terminal and life-limiting illness, and their families.

Index keyword: Childcare

Reading Cygnets Swimming Club for the Mentally Handicapped

c/o 24 Lockstite Way
Goring-on-Thames
Reading
RG8 0AL

Helpline tel: **01734 722522**
Admin tel: 01491 873237
Admin tel: 01491 873237

[C] [✋] [☎]

Description: This is a swimming club for mentally handicapped people. It caters both for competitive swimming and for swimmers who are less able.

Index keyword: Mental Health/Illness

Red Black White

47 Old Hinckley Road
Nuneaton
Warwickshire
CV10 0AA

Helpline tel: **01203 353343**
Admin tel: 01203 353343
Admin fax: 01203 353343

[C] [☎] [NEWS]

Description: Treats children under the age of 18 years suffering from PWS and other birth-marks, where treatment is not readily available on the NHS.

Index keyword: Skin Problems

Reflex Anoxic Seizure Information and Support Group

PO Box 175
Stratford-upon-Avon
Warwickshire
CV37 8YD

Helpline tel: **01789 450564**
Admin tel: 01789 450564
Admin fax: 01789 450564
E-mail: trudie@stars.org.uk

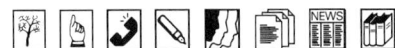

[🌳] [✋] [☎] [✏] [👣] [📋] [NEWS] [📖]

Description: Aims to help and reassure parents of children with RAS; to act as a support group; to bring about more public awareness of RAS; to gather more information to aid research into RAS. Offers links with similarly affected families; information and reports on RAS; video; understanding and friendship among parents.

Index keyword: General Information

Reflexology Information Centre

PO Box 131
Research House
Fraser Road, Greenford
Middlesex
UB6 7DX

Helpline tel: **020 8810 5644**
Admin tel: 020 8810 5644
Admin fax: 020 8810 5645

[☎] [NEWS] [📖]

Description: Offers mainly information on education and training in reflexology, massage and aromatherapy, leading to career practitioners/therapists. Information is available from the practitioners' register on practitioners in various areas.

Index keyword: Complementary Medicine

Registered Nursing Home Association

Calthorpe House
Hagley Road
Edgbaston
Birmingham
B16 8QT

Helpline tel: **0121 454 2511**
Admin tel: 0121 454 2511
Admin fax: 0121 454 0932
Website: www.rnha.co.uk
E-mail: rnhaho@aol.com

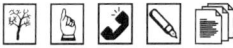

Description: This is a trade association for nursing home owners. Provides an annual reference book listing all nursing homes.

Index keyword: Nursing Homes

RELATE

Herbert Gray College
Little Church Street
Rugby
CV21 3AP

Helpline tel: **01372 464100**
Admin tel: 01788 573241
Admin fax: 01788 535007

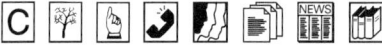

Description: RELATE offers counselling and psychosexual therapy to people who seek advice with adult couple relationships, whether they are married or not. Local centres throughout England, Wales and Northern Ireland can be found in Yellow Pages or local telephone directories under Marriage Guidance or RELATE.

Index keyword: Marriage

Relatives Association, The

5 Tavistock Place
London
WC1H 9SN

Helpline tel: **020 7916 6055**
Admin tel: 020 7692 4302
Admin fax: 020 7916 6093
Opening times: 10.00am–12.30pm and 1.30pm–5.00pm, Mon–Fri

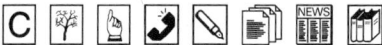

Description: This is a mutual aid organisation of relatives and friends of older people in residential and nursing homes and long-stay hospitals. We offer support and information on choosing a home, paying fees, about care and involving families and friends in Homes.

Index keyword: Elderly:
Accommodation/Housing

Relaxation for Living Trust, The

12 New Street
Chipping Norton
Oxon
OX7 5LJ

Helpline tel: **01608 646100**
Admin tel: 01608 646100
Admin fax: 01608 646100

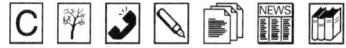

Description: Aims to promote the teaching of physical relaxation. Offers small group classes around the UK; a correspondence course; university-accredited training courses for relaxation teachers; seminars/workshops for business and organisations. Send A5 sae for information.

Index keyword: Complementary Medicine

REMAP GB (Technical Equipment for Disabled People)

'Hazeldene'
Ightham
Sevenoaks
Kent
TN15 9AD

Admin tel: 01732 883818
Admin fax: 01732 886238

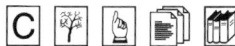

Description: Designs, manufactures and supplies technical aids for disabled people where nothing suitable is available commercially.

Index keyword: Disability: Equipment

RESCARE (The National Society for Mentally Handicapped People in Residential Care)

Rayner House
23 Higher Hillgate
Stockport
Cheshire
SK1 3ER

Helpline tel: **0161 474 7323**
Admin tel: 0161 474 7323
Admin fax: 0161 480 3668
Website: www.rescare.org.uk
E-mail: office@rescare.org.uk

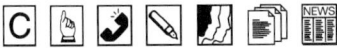

Description: Promotes the relief and welfare of people with a mental handicap in all types of residential care, including the family home. They seek a wide range of residential options, including residential and village communities, and their evolution within suitable hospital sites.

Index keyword: Mental Health/Illness

Restricted Growth Association

PO Box 18
Rugeley
Staffordshire
WS15 2GH

Admin tel: 01889 576571

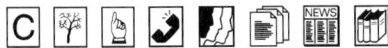

Description: The objectives of the RGA are to remove the substantial social barriers experienced by individuals of restricted growth; to improve the quality of life and help to alleviate the fear and distress experienced by families when their child of restricted growth is born. The association provides information on various aspects of day-to-day living.

Index keyword: General Information

RICA

2 Marylebone Road
London
NW1 4DF

Admin tel: 020 7830 7508
Admin fax: 020 7830 7679

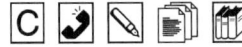

Description: Originally set up by Consumers' Association in 1961, RICA is an independent charity. RICA carries out research and publishes unbiased information on products and services – but concentrates on the special needs of consumers who are elderly or disabled.

Index keyword: Elderly: General Information

Richard Willson Accessible Transport Services

49 Carne View Road
Probus
Truro
Cornwall
TR2 4HZ

Helpline tel: **01726 883460**
Admin tel: 01726 883460
Admin fax: 01726 883460
E-mail: richard.willson@lineone.co.uk
Opening times: All day until 10.00pm

Description: Their principal function is to provide specialised transport for people unable to use conventional transport. Moves people in a conventional hospital bed, by stretcher, wheelchair, or seated and can also offer free advice. Operates throughout mainland Britain, providing long-distance transport.

Index keyword: Disability: General Information

RESCARE (The National Society for Mentally Handicapped People in Residential Care)–Richard Willson Accessible Transport Services

171

Richmond Fellowship

8 Addison Road
London
W14 8DJ

Helpline tel: **020 7603 6373**
Admin tel: 020 7603 6373
Admin fax: 020 7602 8652

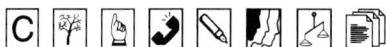

Description: This national charity and housing association runs over 60 projects in the UK. Provides care in the field of mental health and addiction in both long and short stay residential facilities. Also runs workschemes, day centres etc, and provides training and consultancy services for its staff and others in mental health/human relations field.

Index keyword: Mental Health/Illness

RNIB (Northern Ireland)

40 Linenhall Street
Belfast
BT2 8BA

Helpline tel: **028 9032 9373**
Admin tel: 028 9032 9373
Admin fax: 028 9043 9118
Website: www.rnib.org.uk

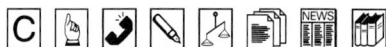

Description: The RNIB Northern Ireland Service Bureau, the RNIB Mobile Resource Unit and the RNIB Sensory Support Service, Londonderry, offer products and services to the visually impaired community in Northern Ireland. Sole agents for British Wireless for the Blind Fund. RNIB Through Windows provides IT for visually impaired students.

Index keyword: Blindness/Visual Handicap

RNIB Multiple Disability Services

7 The Square
111 Broad Street
Edgbaston
Birmingham
B15 1AS

Admin tel: 0121 643 9912
Admin fax: 0121 643 1738
E-mail: mgray@rnib.org.uk

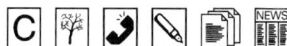

Description: Provides training, by short courses and local programmes of modular training, to paid carers and/or relatives of adults with multiple disability in residential or day care settings.

Index keyword: Disability: General Information

RNIB Talking Book Service

Mount Pleasant
Wembley
Middlesex
HA0 1RR

Admin tel: 020 8903 6666
Admin fax: 020 8903 6916

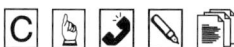

Description: Provides a postal library service for blind and partially-sighted people, of any age, offering a wide range of professionally recorded books on special easy-to-use playback equipment. There is an annual membership subscription, often paid by local authorities. The service covers the whole of the British Isles.

Index keyword: Blindness/Visual Handicap

RNIB Transcription Centre Northwest

67 High Street
Tarporley
Cheshire
CW6 0DP

Helpline tel: **01829 732115**
Admin tel: 01829 732115
Admin fax: 01829 732408
Website: www.rnib.org.uk
E-mail: tarpoley@rnib.org.uk
Opening times: 8.45am–5pm

Description: Part of Royal National Institute for the Blind, works for visually impaired students and people at work in the Northwest and Wales who send study or work texts which they need to read. They then transcribe them to the medium of choice, ie audio cassette, braille, large print.

Index keyword: Blindness/Visual Handicap

RNID Tinnitus Helpline

Castle Cavendish Works
Norton Street
Radford
Nottingham
NG7 5PN

Helpline tel: **0808 8086666**
Admin tel: 0115 942 1520
Admin fax: 0115 978 5012
Website: www.rnid.org.uk
E-mail: tinnitushelpline@btinternet.com
Opening times: 10.00am–3.00pm, Mon–Fri

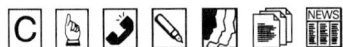

Description: Helps people who experience noises in the ears or head, their families and friends, and the professionals who work with them.

Index keyword: Hearing Problems/ Deafness

Road Peace

PO Box 2579
London
NW10 3PW

Helpline tel: **020 8964 1021**
Admin tel: 020 8964 9353
Admin fax: 020 8138 5103
E-mail: info@roadpeace.org.uk

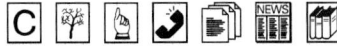

Description: Provides emotional and practical road support to bereaved and injured road traffic victims. Promotes public awareness of danger on the roads and encourages every effort to reduce that danger. Helps victims through the complex and confusing procedures following road death or injury.

Index keyword: General Information

Royal Agricultural Benevolent Institution

Shaw House
27 West Way
Oxford
OX2 0QH

Helpline tel: **01865 724931**
Admin tel: 01865 724931
Admin fax: 01865 202025
Website: www.rabi.org.uk

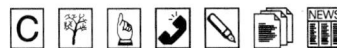

Description: RABI is the national organisation for assisting retired, disabled and other disadvantaged farmers, farm workers, farm managers and their families.

Index keyword: General Information

Royal Air Force Benelovent Fund

67 Portland Place
London
W1N 4AR

Admin tel: 020 7580 8343
Admin fax: 020 7636 7005

C ✋

Description: The fund's purpose is the relief, usually by financial loan or grant, of distress among serving and former members of the Royal Air Force, their widows/widowers and dependants. Application for help should be made by letter to 67 Portland Place.

Index keyword: Ex-Servicemen

Royal Association for Disability And Rehabilitation (RADAR)

12 City Forum
250 City Road
London
EC1V 8AF

Helpline tel: 020 7250 3222
Admin tel: 020 7250 3222
Admin fax: 020 7250 0212
Website: www.radar.org.uk
E-mail: radar@radar.org.uk

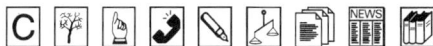

C 🌳 ✋ ☎ ✏ 🦶 ⚗ 📄 NEWS 📊

Description: Campaigns for disabled people's rights and full integration into society. Information and advisory service; active in fields of employment, mobility, housing, holidays, social service provision, social security, education and civil rights, employment, training and transport provision.

Index keyword: Disability: General Information

Royal Association in Aid of Deaf people

27 Old Oak Road
Acton
London
W3 7HN

Helpline tel: 01206 509509
Admin tel: 020 8743 6187
Admin fax: 020 8740 6551

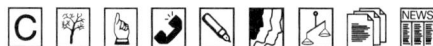

C 🌳 ✋ ☎ ✏ 🦶 ⚗ 📄 NEWS

Description: RAD is committed to meeting the individual needs of people affected by deafness, through its centres situated in south-east England. RAD provides services which include: advocacy, chaplaincy, counselling, information, interpreting, leisure facilities and support groups.

Index keyword: Hearing Problems/ Deafness

Royal British Legion, The

48 Pall Mall
London
SW1Y 5JY

Helpline tel: 0345 725725
Admin tel: 020 7973 7200
Admin fax: 020 7973 7399

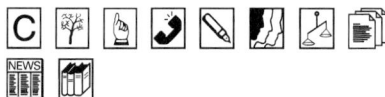

C 🌳 ✋ ☎ ✏ 🦶 ⚗ 📄 NEWS 📊

Description: Britain's premier ex-service organisation for the welfare of ex-servicemen, women and their dependants provides financial assistance, residential and convalescent homes, employment for the disabled, small business advice and loans, resettlement training, free pensions advice, and much more, all financed from public support. Also provides social focus.

Index keyword: Ex-Servicemen

Royal College of Psychiatrists

17 Belgrave Square
London
SW1X 8PG

Helpline tel: **020 7235 2351**
Admin tel: 020 7235 2351
Admin fax: 020 7245 1231
Website: www.rcpsych.ac.uk
E-mail: rcpsych@rcpsych.ac.uk

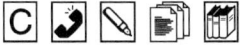

Description: Advances the science and practice of psychiatry and further public education therein to promote study and research into psychiatry and in disciplines connected with the understanding and treatment of mental disorder.

Index keyword: Mental Health/Illness

Royal Gardeners' Orphan Fund, The

48 St Albans Road
Codicote
Hitchin
Hertfordshire
SG4 8UT

Helpline tel: **01438 820783**
Admin tel: 01438 820783

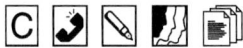

Description: Offers assistance to needy children, not necessarily orphaned, whose parents are employed full-time in horticulture. Gives regular allowances or grants for special, especially educational, purposes.

Index keyword: Gardening

Royal National Institute for Deaf People (Head Office)

19–23 Featherstone Street
London
EC1Y 8SL

Admin tel: 020 7296 8000
Admin fax: 020 7296 8199
Website: www.rnid.org.uk
E-mail: helpline@rnid.org.uk

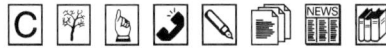

Description: The Organisation runs a regional information service, deaf awareness training, interpreting services and residential centres. They also run Typetalk (the National Telephone Relay Service), the Tinnitus Helpline and test/develop assistive devices.

Index keyword: Hearing Problems/Deafness

Royal National Institute for Deaf People (Northern Ireland)

Wilton House
5 College Square North
Belfast
Northern Ireland
BT1 6AR

Helpline tel: **028 9032 9738**
Admin tel: 028 9032 9738
Admin fax: 028 9031 2032

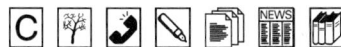

Description: The RNID is the largest voluntary organisation in the UK representing deaf, deafened, hard of hearing and deafblind people. Their vision is for deaf people to exercise their right to full citizenship and to enjoy equal opportunities. The services provided are information, residential care, training, specialist telephone services, communication support and assistive services.

Index keyword: Hearing Problems/ Deafness

Royal National Institute for Deaf People, The (RNID) (Regional Office)

39 Store Street
London
WC1E 7DB

Helpline tel: **020 7813 2480**
Admin tel: 020 7916 4144
Admin fax: 020 7916 4546

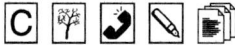

Description: The RNID is the largest charity in the field of deafness and deafblind issues. Regional information service; residential care for deaf people with additional needs; a growing national network of communication support units which provide interpreters and other communication support; deaf awareness training and interpreter training; Typetalk – the national telephone relay service; and the development, testing and marketing of assistive devices.

Index keyword: Hearing Problems/ Deafness

Royal National Institute for the Blind

224 Great Portland Street
London
W1N 6AA

Helpline tel: **020 7388 1266**
Admin tel: 020 7388 1266
Admin fax: 020 7388 2034

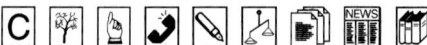

Description: Campaigns for blind and partially-sighted people to enjoy the same rights, freedoms and responsibilities and quality of life as people who are fully sighted. The task of RNIB is to challenge the disabling effects of blindness by providing services to help people determine their own lives; to challenge society's actions, attitudes and assumptions and to challenge the underlying causes of blindness by helping to prevent, cure and alleviate it.

Index keyword: Blindness/Visual Handicap

Royal Orthopaedic Hospital Bone Tumour Service (ROHBTS)

c/o Ward 11, Royal Orthopaedic Hospital
The Woodlands
Bristol Road South, Northfield
Birmingham
B31 2AP

and

The Brick House
Lower Wood Road
Ludlow
Shropshire
SY8 2JQ

Helpline tel: **01584 856209**
Admin tel: 01584 856209
Admin fax: 01584 856648
E-mail: jrichardson17.freeserve.co.uk

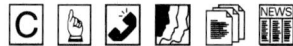

Description: ROHBTS aims to be a support service offering a combination of emotional and practical help. It operates a telephone tree and runs and supports a holiday home for the benefit of patients and immediate family.

Index keyword: Cancer

Royal Society for the Prevention of Accidents

353 Bristol Road
Birmingham
B5 7SL

Helpline tel: **0121 248 2000**
Admin tel: 0121 248 2000
Admin fax: 0121 248 2001
E-mail: help@ROSPA.com

[C] [tree] [phone] [pencil] [leg] [flask] [docs] [NEWS]
[book]

Description: RoSPA aims to exercise a powerful influence for accident prevention, through advice and campaigns. The society provides written and verbal advice, expert witnesses, safety auditing, defensive driving and a range of other training courses; and education of children.

Index keyword: Accident Prevention

Royal Star and Garter Home for Disabled Sailors, Soldiers and Airmen, The

Richmond Hill
Richmond
Surrey
TW10 6RR

Helpline tel: **020 8940 3314**
Admin tel: 020 8940 3314
Admin fax: 020 8940 1953
Opening times: 24 hrs (Nursing Home)

[C] [hand] [phone] [docs]

Description: The Royal Star and Garter Home provides nursing home care and therapy for disabled ex-service men and women.

Index keyword: Ex-Servicemen

S.A.D. (Seasonal Affective Disorder Association)

PO Box 989
Steyning
West Sussex
BN44 3HG

Helpline tel: **01903 814942**
Admin fax: 01903 879939
Website: www.sada.org.uk

[C] [tree] [hand] [pencil] [docs] [NEWS]

Description: Informs health professionals and the public about SAD to provide support for sufferers and their families and to promote research into its causes and treatments.

Index keyword: Seasonal Affective Disorder

Salvation Army

Greig House ADU
20 Garford Street
London
E14 8JG

Helpline tel: **020 7987 5658**
Admin tel: 020 7987 5658
Admin fax: 020 7536 1601
Opening times: 24 hours

[C] [tree] [phone] [leg]

Description: This is a 7–14 day service providing medically supervised detoxification from alcohol. Referrals from any source, but not as a condition of court. Funding by local boroughs and DSS, if relevant, or by private arrangement if employed. Residential. History of minor misuse of other substances not a barrier.

Index keyword: General Information

Salvation Army

Salvation Army Social Services
105–109 Judd Street
Kings Cross
London
WC1H 9TS

Helpline tel: **020 7383 4230**
Admin fax: 020 7383 2562

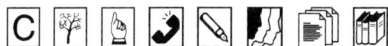

Description: The Salvation Army is an international religious and social welfare movement and a branch of the mainstream Christian church. Its objective is the physical, moral and spiritual regeneration of the people it serves, through the provision of basic human necessities, counselling, living and preaching the Christian Gospel.

Index keyword: General Information

Salvation Army Family Tracing Service, The

105–109 Judd Street
Kings Cross
London
WC1H 9TS

Helpline tel: **020 7383 2772**
Admin tel: 020 7383 2772
Admin fax: 020 7388 2964

Description: The service assists in locating adult members of families.

Index keyword: General Information

Samaritans, The

10 The Grove
Slough
Berks
SL1 1QP

Helpline tel: **0345 909090**
Admin tel: 01753 216500
Admin fax: 01753 819004
Website: www.samaritan.org.uk
E-mail: admin@samaritans.org.uk

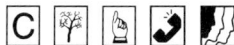

Description: The Samaritans is a registered charity, founded in 1953. The Samaritans is available, 24 hours a day, to provide confidential and emotional support to anyone passing through crisis and at risk of suicide. The Samaritans aims to provide society with a better understanding of suicide and the value of expressing feelings that may lead to suicide.

Index keyword: Counselling

Schizophrenia Association of Great Britain

Bryn Hyfryd
The Crescent
Bangor
Gwynedd
LL57 2AG

Helpline tel: **01248 354048**
Admin tel: 01248 354048
Admin fax: 01248 354048
Website: www.btinternet.com/~sagb
E-mail: sagb@btinternet.com
Opening times: 9.00am–4.00pm, Mon–Thurs; 9.00am–3.15pm, Fri

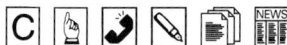

Description: Helps patients suffering from Schizophrenia and their families. Continues research into the causes of Schizophrenia. Educates the public about Schizophrenia and enlists sympathy and support. Two newsletters a year are sent to members. There is a Helpline for information.

Index keyword: Schizophrenia

School of Phytotherapy (Herbal Medicine)

Bucksteep Manor
Bodle Street Green
Nr Hailsham
East Sussex
BN27 4RJ

Helpline tel: **01323 832858**
Admin tel: 01323 833812; 01323 833814
Admin fax: 01323 833869

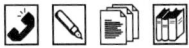

Description: Their training school for practitioners of phytotherapy (herbal medicine) incorporates a four-year BSc (honours) degree course; four-year tutorial/correspondence course; specially structured course for practising general practitioners; plus a one-year basic home study course. Clinical training may be carried out at three training clinics.

Index keyword: Complementary Medicine

Scoliosis Association UK

2 Ivebury Court
325 Latimer Road
London
W10 6RA

Helpline tel: **020 8964 1166**
Admin tel: 020 8964 5343
Admin fax: 020 8964 5343
Website: www.sauk.org.uk
E-mail: sauk.org.uk
Opening times: 10.00am–2.00pm, Mon; 10.00am–5.00pm, Tues–Thurs; 1.00pm–5.00pm, Fri

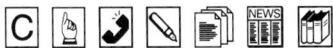

Description: SAUK is the only national support organisation for people with scoliosis. It seeks to spread knowledge about scoliosis, alerting the public and people in contact with children and young people to the need for early detection of scoliosis.

Index keyword: Scoliosis

SCOPE (Cerebral Palsy Helpline)

PO Box 833
Milton Keynes
Bucks
MK12 5NY

Helpline tel: **0808 800 3333**
Admin fax: 01908 321051
Website: www.scope.org.uk
E-mail: cphelpline@scope.org.uk
Opening times: 9.00am–9.00pm, Mon–Fri; 2.00pm–6.00pm, Sat–Sun

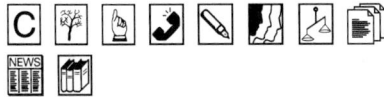

Description: SCOPE provides a range of services for people with cerebral palsy, their families and carers, including schools, residential care, information and careers advice. SCOPE has a helpline, available seven days a week; subscription to a monthly newsletter, 'Disability Now'; six regional offices; and over 250 affiliated local groups.

Index keyword: Cerebral Palsy

Scottish Association for Mental Health

Cumbria House
15 Carlton Court
Glasgow
G5 9JP

Helpline tel: **0141 568 7000**
Admin tel: 0141 568 7000 (9.00am–5.00pm)
Admin fax: 0141 568 7001
E-mail: enquire@samh.org.uk
Opening times: 11.30am–4.30pm, Mon–Fri

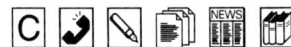

Description: This is a voluntary organisation with many years' experience of providing direct services to people with mental health problems and of campaigning for recognition of their fundamental human and citizen rights.

Index keyword: Mental Health/Illness

Scottish Association for the Deaf, The

Moray House, Institute of Education
Heriot-Watt University
Holyrood Road
Edinburgh
EH8 8AQ

Helpline tel: **0131 558 3390 (text)**
Admin tel: 0131 557 0591
Admin fax: 0131 557 6922

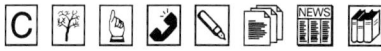

Description: Promotes quality of life for all deaf people in Scotland. Aims to assess the needs of deaf people, to enable deaf people to gain more independence, to obtain greater access for deaf people in all fields of life, to obtain equal opportunities for all deaf people.

Index keyword: Hearing Problems/Deafness

Scottish Association of Health Councils

24A Palmerston Place
Edinburgh
EH12 5AL

Admin tel: 0131 220 4101
Admin fax: 0131 220 4108
E-mail: SAHC@sol.co.uk
Opening times: 9.00am–5.00pm, Mon–Fri

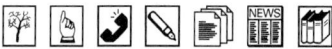

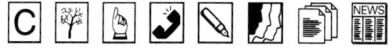

Description: The Association pursues strategies which deliver openness and access to information; public involvement in health matters; equity, access and choice in health services; partnership with the professionals; the empowerment of the user of health services.

Index keyword: General Health

Scottish Cot Death Trust

Royal Hospital for Sick Children
Yorkhill
Glasgow
G3 8SJ

Helpline tel: **0141 357 3946**
Admin tel: 0141 357 3946
Admin fax: 0141 334 1376
E-mail: hblw@clinmed.gla.ac.uk
Opening times: 9.00am–5.00pm, Mon–Fri

Description: Aims to raise funds for research into cot death; to improve support for bereaved parents; to educate the public and healthcare professionals about cot death.

Index keyword: Bereavement

Scottish Council on Alcohol

2nd Floor
166 Buchanan Street
Glasgow
G1 2NH

Admin tel: 0141 333 9677
Admin fax: 0141 333 1606
E-mail: sca@clara.net
Opening times: 9.00am–5.00pm, Mon–Thurs; 9.00am–4.30pm, Fri

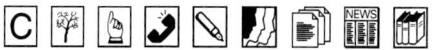

Description: Aims to develop a network of local Councils on Alcohol. Promotes the adoption of safe and sensible drinking styles for people who choose to drink. Works with employers, courts, prisons, statutory agencies, on a national and international basis.

Index keyword: Alcohol Problems

Scottish Down's Syndrome Association

158–160 Balgreen Road
Edinburgh
EH11 3AU

Helpline tel: **0131 313 4225 (24 hours)**
Admin tel: 0131 313 4225
Admin fax: 0131 313 4285
Website: www.sdsa.org.uk
E-mail: info@sdsa.org.uk
Opening times: 9.30am–4.30pm, Mon–Fri

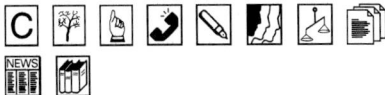

Description: Supports people with Down's Syndrome and their families throughout Scotland.

Index keyword: Down's Syndrome

Scottish Dyslexia Association

Unit 3
Stirling Business Centre
Wellgreen
Stirling
FK8 2DZ

Helpline tel: **01786 446650**
Admin tel: 01786 471235
Admin fax: 01786 471235
E-mail: dyslexia.scotland@dial.pipex.com
Opening times: 9.00am–5.00pm, Mon–Fri

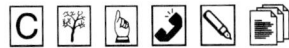

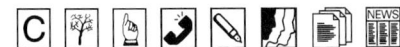

Description: The association seeks to further the knowledge and awareness of dyslexia at national level through contact with statutory bodies, national agencies and other organisations. Local associations throughout Scotland provide help and information for dyslexic children, adults and teachers.

Index keyword: Dyslexia

Scottish Huntington's Association

Thistle House
61 Main Road
Elderslie
PA5 9BA

Helpline tel: **01505 322245**
Admin tel: 01505 322245
Admin fax: 01505 382980
Website: www.hdscotland.org
E-mail: sha-admin@hdscotland.org
Opening times: 9.00am–5.00pm, Mon–Thurs; 9.00am–4.00pm, Fri

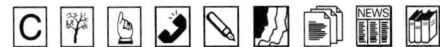

Description: The association offers help and support to people with Huntington's disease, their families and carers. The aim is to provide better services, and to educate professionals and lay people about the condition.

Index keyword: Huntington's Disease

Scottish Motor Neurone Disease Association

Unit 4
76 Firhill Road
Glasgow
G20 7BA

Helpline tel: **0141 945 1077**
Admin tel: 0141 945 1077
Admin fax: 0141 945 2578
Website: www.scotmnd.org.uk
E-mail: info@scotmnd.sol.co.uk
Opening times: 9.00am–5.00pm, Mon–Fri

Description: Aims to help people with motor neurone disease, to advise their carers and families and to finance research into the cause and cure of the disease. Five care advisers cover the whole of Scotland, not only helping patients and families, but also advising community medical staff at all levels.

Index keyword: Motor Neurone Diseases

Scottish Pre-School Play Association

14 Elliot Place
Glasgow
G3 8EP

Admin tel: 0141 221 4141
Admin fax: 0141 221 6043
Opening times: 9.00am–4.30pm, Mon–Fri

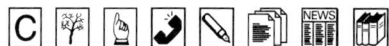

Description: SPPA is a Scottish education charity committed to the development of quality care and education in pre-school groups; it respects the rights, responsibilities and needs of all children and their parents.

Index keyword: Education

Scottish Society for Autism

Hilton House
Alloa Business Park
Whins Road
Alloa
FK10 3SA

Helpline tel: **01259 720044**
Admin tel: 01259 720044
Admin fax: 01259 720051
Website: www.autism-m-scotland.org.uk
E-mail: autism@autism-m-scotland.org.uk
Opening times: 9.00am–5.00pm,
Mon–Thurs; 9.00am–4.30pm, Fri

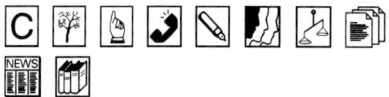

Description: The SSA is the biggest provider of services for autism in Scotland. They operate a residential school for children, training and supported living for young adults, respite care and family support services, training for carers and professionals; support self-help groups and produce an information pack and members' magazine.

Index keyword: Autism

Scottish Spina Bifida Association

190 Queensferry Road
Edinburgh
EH4 2BW

Helpline tel: **08459 111112 (family support services)**
Admin tel: 0131 332 0743
Admin fax: 0131 343 3651
Website:
http://ourworld.compuserve.com/homepages/SSBAhq
E-mail: ssbahq@compuserve.com
Opening times: 9.00am–5.00pm, Mon–Fri

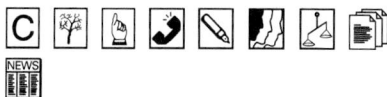

Description: Works to increase public awareness and understanding of people with spina bifida/hydrocephalus and allied disorders. Aims to secure provision for their special needs and those of their family.

Index keyword: Spina Bifida

Scottish Women's Aid

12 Torphichen Street
Edinburgh
EH3 8JQ

Helpline tel: **0131 221 0401**
Admin tel: 0131 221 0481
Admin fax: 0131 221 0402

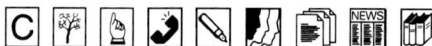

Description: Works with a network of 39 local women's aid groups throughout Scotland to provide services for abused women and their children. Provides training; promotes rights and needs of children who have experienced domestic violence; campaigns and lobbies to raise awareness and improve legislation affecting abused women and their children.

Index keyword: Women's Health

Scout Holiday Homes Trust

Baden-Powell House
Queen's Gate
London
SW7 5JS

Helpline tel: **020 7584 7030**
Admin tel: 020 7590 5152
Admin fax: 020 7590 5103
Opening times: 8.30am–4.00pm, Mon–Fri

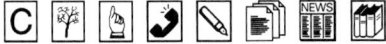

C 🌳 ✍️ 📞 ✏️ 📑 📰 📖

Description: Provides low cost self-catering holidays for families with special needs (families with a disabled member, low income families, elderly, one parent) in their own caravans and chalets on fully commercial holiday sites. You don't have to have a scouting connection.

Index keyboard: Disability: Care Scheme/Holidays

Seeability

56–66 Highlands Road
Leatherhead
Surrey
KT22 8NR

Admin tel: 01372 373086
Admin fax: 01372 370143
E-mail: reception.seeability.org
Opening hours: 24 hours

Description: Aims to provide community, residential and day care for people of 18 and over who are blind with other disabilities, including learning and physical disabilities, head injuries and degenerative diseases; to enable each individual to achieve maximum potential. Also provides visual impairment awareness training for other organisations.

Index keyboard: Blindness/Visual Handicap

Self Help Team, The

20 Pelham Road
Sherwood Rise
Nottingham
NG5 1AP

Helpline tel: **0115 969 1212**
Admin tel: 0115 969 1212
Admin fax: 0115 960 2049

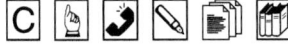

C ✍️ 📞 ✏️ 📑 📖

Description: The Self Help Team provides information about and services for self-help groups in Nottingham. They work directly with self-help groups, interested professionals and the general public. Services offered: information about local groups and national organisations; support to new and existing groups; training and development; promotion of good practice through research and publications.

Index keyboard: General Health

SeniorLine

Help The Aged
St James's Walk
Clerkenwell Green
London
EC1R 0BE

Helpline tel: **0808 800 6565**
Admin tel: 020 7253 0253
Admin fax: 020 7250 4474

C ✍️ 📞 📑

Description: SeniorLine is Help The Aged's national advice and information service. They can provide general advice on issues affecting older people and give details of local or national organisations that may be of use.

Index keyboard: Elderly: General Information

Sense (Northern Ireland)

Knockbracken Healthcare Park
Saintfield Road
Belfast
BT8 8DH

Helpline tel: **01232 705858**
Admin tel: 01232 705858
Admin fax: 01232 705688

[C] [🌳] [👁] [📞] [✏️] [🦵] [⚗️] [📄]
[NEWS] [📖]

Description: Sense works with families,
individuals, carers and professionals on
deafblind issues. Also runs a 10-person
residential home and education and
resource centre at Carrickfergus, County
Antrim.

Index keyboard: Hearing Problems/
Deafness

Sense (The National Deafblind and Rubella Association)

11–13 Clifton Terrace
Finsbury Park
London
N4 3SR

Admin tel: 020 7272 7774
Admin fax: 020 7272 6012
Website: www.sense.org.uk
E-mail: enquiries@sense.org.uk
Opening times: 9.00am–5.30pm, Mon–Fri

[C] [🌳] [👁] [📞] [✏️] [⚗️] [📄] [NEWS] [📖]

Description: Sense is the leading
international organisation providing
services, advice, support and information
for children and young adults who are
deafblind, their families and professionals
in the field. Sense aims to enhance quality
of life for the 23,000 deafblind people in
the UK through campaigning and
providing services for their unique needs.

Index keyboard: Hearing Problems/Deafness

Sequal Trust, The

Ddolhir
Glyn Ceiriog
Llangollen
Clwyd
LL20 7NP

Admin tel: 01691 718331
Admin fax: 01691 718331

[C] [📞] [✏️] [📄] [NEWS]

Description: The trust provides
communication aids on a free loan basis
to severely disabled children and adults
who have little movement and/or speech.

Index keyboard: Disability: General
Information

Seriously Ill for Medical Research (SIMR)

PO Box 504
Dunstable
Bedfordshire
LU6 2LU

Helpline tel: **01582 873108**
Admin tel: 01582 873108
Admin fax: 01582 873705
Website: www.simr.org.uk
E-mail: info@simr.org.uk
Opening times: 9.00am–5.00pm, Mon–Fri

[👁] [⚗️] [📄] [NEWS] [📖]

Description: SIMR is an independent,
voluntary organisation, formed to
promote research into crippling,
debilitating and progressive diseases and
to support the humane use of animals in
medical research.

Index keyword: General Information

Sesame Institute UK

Christchurch
27 Blackfriars Road
London
SE1 8NY

Helpline tel: **020 7633 9690**
Admin tel: 020 7633 9690
E-mail: seasameinstituteuk@btinternet.com
Opening times: 10.00am–4.00pm, Tues,
Thurs, Fri

Description: Offers training for students
in drama and movement therapy;
professional support and membership for
practitioners; liaison between
practitioners and institutions and
therapies; information and short courses;
fundraising.

Index keyword: General Information

SHARE Community Ltd

64 Altenberg Gardens
London
SW11 1JL

Admin tel: 020 7924 2949
Admin fax: 020 7350 1625
Opening hours: 9.00am–5.00pm, Mon–Fri

Description: SHARE Community Ltd is a
training and rehabilitation centre for
disabled adults, covering all forms of
disability and related problems. Training
consists of four courses, namely Business
Administration, Information Technology,
Catering, Horticulture. These courses are
taught to NVQ1 level.

Index keyword: Disability: General
Information

Shared Care Network

The Norah Fry Research Centre
3 Priory Road
Bristol
BS8 1TX

Admin tel: 0117 946 7230
Admin fax: 0117 973 1142
E-mail: shared-care@bristol.ac.uk
Opening times: 9.00am–5.00pm, Mon–Fri

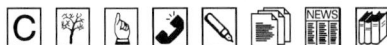

Description: Shared Care Network is the
umbrella organisation for approximately
300 services in England and Northern
Ireland which links disabled children and
their families with host families who are
willing to offer occasional care. Gives
advice to carers, professionals and
parents on short-term care facilities and
regional organisations. Also publishes a
directory of schemes, surveys etc and
organises conferences and training
events.

Index keyword: Disability: Care Scheme/
Holidays

Shelter

88 Old Street
London
EC1V 9HU

Helpline tel: **0808 800 4444**
Admin fax: 020 7505 2169
Website: www.shelter.org.uk
E-mail: info@shelter.org.uk
Opening times: Mon–Fri, 24 hours

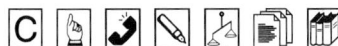

Description: Shelter provides free,
independent housing advice through a
national network of housing aid centres,
and a national 24 hr freephone emergency
advice service called Shelterline. Shelter
combines practical help with
campaigning on behalf of homeless and
badly housed people towards a fairer

housing system to make affordable permanent housing available to everybody.

Index keyword: Homelessness

Shingles Support Society

41 North Road
London
N7 9DP

Helpline tel: **020 7607 9061**
Admin tel: 020 7607 9661
E-mail: herpes.virusesassociation.virgin.net
Opening times: 10.00am–8.00pm, Mon–Fri

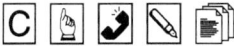

C 👆 📞 🖊 📑

Description: Supplies information and advice on medical treatment and self-help for post-herpetic neuralgia (PHN) which, particularly in older patients, can follow shingles.

Index keyword: Herpes

Shipwrecked Mariners' Society

1 North Pallant
Chichester
West Sussex
PO19 1TL

Helpline tel: **01243 787761**
Admin tel: 01243 789329
Admin fax: 01243 530853
Opening times: 9.15am–4.30pm, Mon–Fri

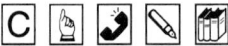

C 👆 📞 🖊 📚

Description: Aims to relieve distress among the seafaring community by making discretionary financial grants to former mariners and fishermen and to their widows. Also provides immediate financial aid to dependants of seamen lost at sea and aid to seamen shipwrecked on the coasts of the British Isles.

Index keyword: General Information

Sickle Cell and Thalassaemia Unit (City and Hackney)

Homerton Hospital
Homerton Row
London
E9 6SR

Helpline tel: **020 8510 7313**
Admin tel: 020 8919 7313
Admin fax: 020 8510 7323
Opening times: 9.00am–5.00pm, Mon–Fri

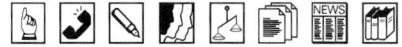

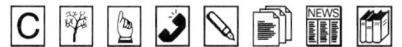

👆 📞 🖊 👣 📐 📑 NEWS 📚

Description: Provides education, counselling, welfare support, community support, screening, training, health promotion, awareness-raising and research.

Index keyword: Sickle Cell/Thalassaemia

Sickle Cell Society

54 Station Road
Harlesden
London
NW10 4UA

Helpline tel: **020 8961 7795**
Admin tel: 020 8961 7795; 020 8961 4006
Admin fax: 020 8961 8346
Website: www.sicklecellsociety.org
E-mail: sicklecellsoc@btinternet.com
Opening times: 9.00am–5.00pm, Mon–Fri

C 🌳 👆 📞 🖊 📑 NEWS 📚

Description: The Sickle Cell Society provides support to sickle cell sufferers and their families. It promotes awareness of the disorder via newsletter, information leaflets, books, videos and by giving talks. The Society offers financial assistance in the form of welfare and educational grants, and provides holiday and recreational activities.

Index keyboard: Sickle Cell/Thalassaemia

Sickle Watch (UK)

West Indian Cultural Centre
9 Clarendon Road
London
N8 0DJ

Helpline tel: **020 8888 2148**
Admin tel: 020 8888 2148
Admin fax: 020 8881 5204
E-mail: neville.claire@cw.com.net
Opening hours: 9.00am–5.00pm, Mon–Fri

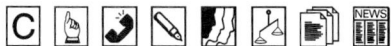

[icons]

Description: Aims to raise the level of awareness of sickle cell disorder by way of publications, lectures, etc; to raise funds to sponsor promising areas of research; to establish a database of research material for professionals and students.

Index keyboard: Sickle Cell/ Thalassaemia

Sight Savers International

Grosvenor Hall
Bolnore Road
Haywards Heath
West Sussex
RH16 4BX

Admin tel: 01444 446600
Admin fax: 01444 446688
Website: www.sightsavers.org.uk
E-mail: enquiry@sightsaversint.org.uk
Opening times: 9.00am–5.00pm, Mon–Fri

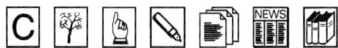

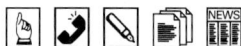

[icons]

Description: Sight Savers International supports eyecare, blindness prevention, education and rehabilitation programmes in over 20 developing countries.

Index keyboard: Blindness/Visual Handicap

Single Parent Action Network

Millpond
Lower Ashley Road
Easton
Bristol
BS5 0XJ

Helpline tel: **0117 951 4231**
Admin tel: 0117 951 4231
Admin fax: 0117 935 5208
Website: www.spanuk.org.uk
E-mail: spanuk@netgates.co.uk
Opening times: 9.00am–5.00pm, Mon–Fri

[icons]

Description: SPAN is a national, multiracial organisation which works to improve policies and practice for single parents and their children, and to support self-help groups in different parts of the country. We offer individual single parents advice and information.

Index keyboard: Childcare

Single Parent Travel Club

37 Sunningdale Park
Queen Victoria Road
New Tupton
Chesterfield
S42 6DZ

Helpline tel: **01246 865069**
Admin tel: 01246 865069

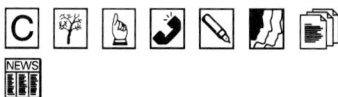

[icons]

Description: Organises low cost weekend breaks and holidays and has a network of local groups throughout Britain.

Index keyboard: Holidays

Skill (National Bureau for Students with Disabilities)

Chapter House
18–20 Crucifix Lane
London
SE1 3JW

Helpline tel: **0800 328 5050**
Admin tel: 0800 328 5050
Admin fax: 020 7450 0650
Website: www.skills.org.uk
E-mail: skillnetburbis@compuserve.com
Opening times: 1.30pm–4.30pm, Mon–Fri
minicom: 0800 0682422

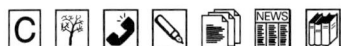

Description: Skill helps young people and adults with any type of disability to realise their potential. Works in further and higher education, training and employment throughout the UK. Provides telephone advice and information to anyone involved in education.

Index keyboard: Disability: General Information

Smith-Magenis Syndrome Foundation

42 Blackmore Road
Malvern
Worcs
WR14 1ZT

Helpline tel: **01684–566606**
Contact: Yolanda Campbell

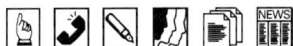

Description: Collates and distributes information and promotes awareness of Smith-Magenis Syndrome. Enables families with similar problems and experiences to contact each other for mutual support.

Index keyboard: Smith-Magenis Syndrome

Smokeline (Scotland)

Network Scotland
The Mews
57 Ruthven Lane
Glasgow
G12 9JA

Helpline tel: **0800 848484**
Opening times: 12.00
(noon)–12.00(midnight) – 7 days

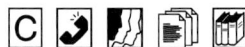

Description: Smokeline provides support and encouragement to people wishing to stop smoking or who have recently stopped and want to stay stopped. Callers can receive a free booklet, *You can stop smoking*. Calls are free and confidential.

Index keyboard: Smoking

Snowdon Award Scheme

22 Horsham Court
6 Brighton Road
Horsham
West Sussex
RH13 5BA

Admin tel: 01403 211252
Admin fax: 01403 271553
Website:
http://.members@aol.com/snowaward
E-mail: snowaward@aol.com
Opening times: 9.00am–5.00pm, Mon–Fri

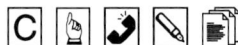

Description: The Snowdon Awards are based on a trust fund set up by the Earl of Snowdon to provide bursaries which enable physically disabled young people (17–25) to pursue opportunities for further education or training.

Index keyword: Disability: General Information

Society for Horticultural Therapy

Goulds Ground
Vallis Way
Frome
Somerset
BA 11 3DW

Helpline tel: **01373 467072**
Admin tel: 01373 464782
Admin fax: 01373 464782
Opening times: Visually impaired only

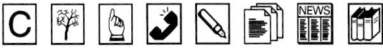

C 🌳 👆 📞 ✏️ 📑 📰 📚

Description: Promotes and supports the use of gardening to improve the quality of life for people with all kind of needs.

Index keyword: Gardening

Society for Mucopolysaccharide Diseases, The

46 Woodside Road
Amersham
Buckinghamshire
HP6 5AJ

Helpline tel: **07712 653 258**
Admin tel: 01494 434156
Admin fax: 01494 434252
Website:
http://home.btconnect.com/mps
E-mail: mps@btconnect.com
Opening times: 9.00am–5.00pm, Mon–Fri

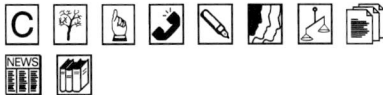

C 🌳 👆 📞 ✏️ 🦶 ⚗️ 📑 📰 📚

Description: The society provides support to families whose children have a mucopolysaccharide or related disease. There are 12 regional support groups in UK; annual conference; advocacy service in housing, welfare benefits and education.

Index keyword: Children: General Information

Society for the Autistically Handicapped (SFTAH)

199–201 Blandford Avenue
Kettering
Northamptonshire
NN16 9AT

Helpline tel: **01536 523274**
Admin tel: 01536 523274
Admin fax: 01536 523274

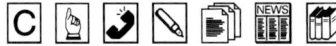

C 👆 📞 ✏️ 📑 📰 📚

Description: The society exists to increase awareness of autism and of both well established and newly developed approaches in the diagnosis, assessment, handling and treatment of people suffering from autism.

Index keyword: Austism

Society for the Protection of Unborn Children

5–6 St Matthew Street
London
SW1P 2JT

Helpline tel: **0845 603 8501 (7 days; 7pm–10pm)**
Admin tel: 020 7222 5845
Admin fax: 020 7222 0630
Website: www.spuc.org.uk
E-mail: enquiry@spuc.org.uk
Opening times: 9.00am–5.30pm, Mon–Fri

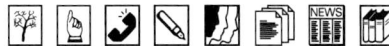

🌳 👆 📞 ✏️ 🦶 📑 📰 📚

Description: Defends and promotes the life of unborn children and the welfare of mothers before and after birth. It provides post-abortion counselling; and defends the right to live of the disabled, born and unborn.

Index keyword: Pregnancy and Childbirth

Society of Chiropodists and Podiatrists

53 Welbeck Street
London
W1M 7HE

Admin tel: 020 7486 3381
Admin fax: 020 7935 6359
Website: www.feetforlife.org
E-mail: eng@scpod.org
Opening times: 9.00am–5.00pm, Mon–Fri

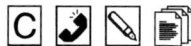

Description: The Society of Chiropodists and Podiatrists is the professional association for state registered chiropodists. To become state registered, it is necessary to undertake a three-year degree course, and only state registered chiropodists may work in the NHS. Make sure your chiropodist is state registered (SRCh).

Index keyword: Feet

Soil Association

Bristol House
40–56 Victoria Street
Bristol
BS1 6DY

Admin tel: 0117 914 2444
Admin fax: 0117 925 2504
Website: www.soilassociation.org
E-mail: info@soilassociation.org
Opening times: 9.00am–5.30pm, Mon–Fri

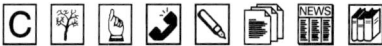

Description: Aims to research, develop and promote sustainable relationships between soils, plants, animals, people and the biosphere, in order to produce healthy foods and other products whilst protecting and enhancing the environment. Certification of organic food and farming and sustainable forestry, and promotion of local food links.

Index keyword: Environmental Health

Soldiers', Sailors' and Airmen's Families Association

Queen Elizabeth The Queen Mother House
19 Queen Elizabeth Street
London
SE1 2LP

Helpline tel: **020 7403 8783**
Admin tel: 020 7403 8783
Admin fax: 020 7403 8815
Opening times: 9.15am–5.00pm, Mon–Fri

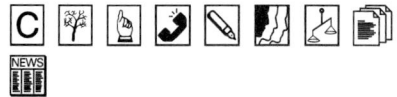

Description: The aim of the association is to look after the welfare of service and ex-service people and their families and dependants through an extensive branch network and thousands of volunteers. Help may be of an advisory, financial or practical nature, or it may be friendship.

Index keyword: Ex-Servicemen

Solemates

46 Gordon Road
Chingford
London
E4 6BU

Helpline tel: **020 8524 2423**
Admin tel: 020 8524 2423
Opening times: 9.00am–5.00pm, Mon–Fri

Description: This is a partnering service for people with odd-sized feet (or only one foot). Information on where to obtain odd-sized footwear throughout the British Isles.

Index keyword: Disability: Equipment

SOS Talisman

21 Grays Corner
Ley Street
Ilford
Essex
IG2 7RQ

Admin tel: 020 8554 5579
Admin fax: 020 8554 1090

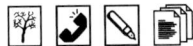

Description: SOS Talisman are distributors of identification jewellery.

Index keyword: General Information

Speakeasy (Association of Speech Impaired)

34 Newark Street
London
E1 2AA

Helpline tel: 020 7377 7177
Admin tel: 020 7377 7177
Admin fax: 020 7377 7177

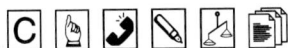

Description: Aims to provide a network of support and advice; to improve public and service providers' awareness of communication impairment; to provide services.

Index keyword: Speech Difficulties

Special Families Trust

Erme House
Station Road
Plympton
Plymouth
Devon
PL7 2AU

Helpline tel: 01752 347577
Admin tel: 01752 346861
Admin fax: 01752 344611

Website: www.mywebpage.net/special-families
E-mail: specialfamiliestrust@care4free.net

Description: Is a free service for physically disabled people, their families and their carers worldwide. Members are able to swap their specially adapted homes with each other for weekend breaks, full holiday swaps or 'come and stay' breaks, confident that their needs will be met as in their own homes.

Index keyword: Disabled/Families/Carers

Spinal Injuries Association

76 St James's Lane
London
N10 3DF

Helpline tel: 0800 980 00501
Admin tel: 020 8444 2121
Admin fax: 020 8444 3761
Website: www.spinal.co.uk
E-mail: sia@spinal.co.uk
Opening times: 9.30am–1.00pm and 2.00pm–5.30pm, Mon–Fri

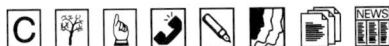

Description: SIA is a self-help group controlled and run by spinal cord injured people to assist those with similar disabilities to get back to an ordinary life. It offers an information service, a confidential welfare service, a care attendant agency and advice on holidays.

Index keyword: Spinal Injuries

Spinal Injuries Scotland (SIS)

Festival Business Centre
150 Brand Street
Glasgow
G51 1DH

Helpline tel: **0141 314 0057**
Admin tel: 0141 314 0056
Admin fax: 0141 314 0082
Website: www.sisonline.org
E-mail: info@sisonline.org
Opening times: 9.00am–5.00pm, Mon–Fri

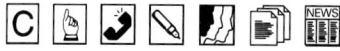

Description: SIS is a registered charity which offers support and information for all spinal cord injured in Scotland, by means of telephone counselling service, information service on holidays, equipment, etc. SIS promotes sport as part of rehabilitation and will actively support sport for tetraplegics.

Index keyword: Spinal Injuries

St John Ambulance

I Grosvenor Crescent
London
SW1X 7EF

Helpline tel: **020 7235 5231**
Admin tel: 020 7235 5231
Admin fax: 020 7235 0796
Website: www.sja.org.uk
E-mail: postmaster@nhgsja.org.uk
Opening times: 8.00am–5.30pm

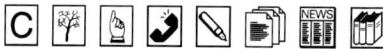

Description: Provides First Aid training nationwide, First Aid, care in the community and a nationwide library service.

Index keyword: First Aid

St Vincent de Paul Society (England and Wales)

14 Blandford Street
London
W1V 4DR

Helpline tel: **020 7935 9126**
Admin fax: 020 7935 9136
Website: http://come.to/SVP
E-mail: svpuk@btconnect.com

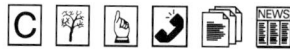

Description: Main activities involve personal visitation to the needy in their homes and in institutions, particularly the lonely, sick and aged. Modest material aid may be given in certain cases. Referrals through head office. Also run a number of projects – furniture units, childrens camps and help with holidays for needy people.

Index keyword: General Information

Standing Conference On Drug Abuse (SCODA)

32–36 Loman Street
London SE1 OEE

Helpline tel: **020 7928 9500**
Admin tel: 020 7928 9500
Admin fax: 020 7928 3343
Opening hours: 10.00am–4.30pm

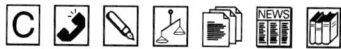

Description: SCODA seeks to reduce the harmful effects of drug use through informed debate, and through the promotion of best practice and effective, comprehensive services. It is an independent membership organisation, providing a voice for drug services and others concerned about the effects of drug use on individuals and communities.

Index keyword: Drug Addiction/Side Effects

Steroid Aid Group

PO Box 220
London
E17 3JR

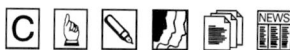

Description: Provides advice and information on cortico steroids. Produces three newsletters per annum and publishes details of steroid side effects for doctors.

Index keyword: Steroids

Stillbirth And Neonatal Death Society (SANDS)

28 Portland Place
London
W1N 4DE

Helpline tel: **020 7436 5881**
Admin tel: 020 7436 7940
Admin fax: 020 7436 3715
Website: www.uk-sands.org
E-mail: support@uk-sands.org

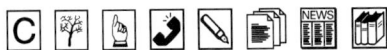

Description: Offers support, through self-help groups and befriending, to people bereaved by pregnancy loss, stillbirth and neonatal death. Also aims to encourage better awareness within the health profession and general public of the feelings and needs of bereaved parents.

Index keyword: Bereavement

Streetwise Youth

11 Eardley Crescent
London
SW5 9JS

Helpline tel: **020 7370 0406**
Admin tel: 020 7370 0406
Admin fax: 020 7244 0037
Website: www.swy@dircon.co.uk
E-mail: swy@dircon.co.uk
Opening times: 4.00pm–7.00pm (Mon); 12.30pm–4.00pm (Wed–Fri), appointment at other times

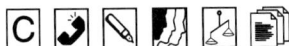

Description: Streetwise Youth provides a confidential advice, information and support service to young men, aged 25

and under, who are involved in selling sex. The aim is to promote their well-being and enable them to make informed choices about their lives.

Index keyword: Children: General Information

Stroke Association, The

CHSA House
123–127 Whitecross Street
London
EC1Y 8JJ

Helpline tel: **0845 3033 100**
Admin tel: 020 7566 0300
Admin fax: 020 7490 2686
Website: www.stroke.org.uk
E-mail: stroke@stroke.org.uk
Opening times: 9.00am–5.00pm, Mon–Fri

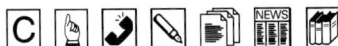

Description: Supports research and health education towards the prevention of stroke; provides direct help for stroke people and their families through its community and welfare services.

Index keyword: Stroke

Sturge-Weber Foundation (UK)

Burleigh
348 Pinhoe Road
Exeter
EX4 8AF

Helpline tel: **01392 464675**
Admin tel: 01392 464675
Admin fax: 01392 464675
Website: www.sturgeweber.org.uk
E-mail: support@sturgeweber.org.uk
Opening times: 24 hours

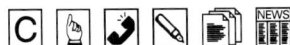

Description: The Foundation exists to support sufferers and their families and to raise public awareness of this condition. Sturge-Weber clinic at Great Ormond Street. Family week-end once a year.

Index keyword: General Information

Sudden Death Support Association

Chapel Green House
Chapel Green
Wokingham
Berkshire
RG40 3ER

Helpline tel: **01189 790790**
Admin fax: 01189 790790

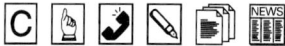

C 👆 📞 ✏️ 📑 📰

Description: The Association is run by people who have themselves lost someone under sudden or tragic circumstances. They offer support and help to people recently bereaved in similar circumstances.

Index keyword: Bereavement

Support Organisation For Trisomy (UK) (SOFT)

48 Froggatts Ride
Walmley
Sutton Coldfield
West Midlands
B76 2TQ

Admin tel: 0121 351 3122
Admin fax: 01989 567480
Website: www.soft.org.uk

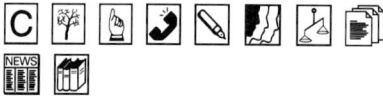

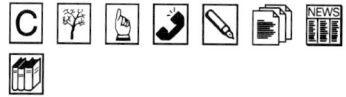

C 🌳 👆 📞 ✏️ 🦶 📑 📰 📊

Description: Supports more than 350 families affected by Edwards' Syndrome and Patau's Syndrome. Offers help and support in feeding, caring, pre-natal care and bereavement counselling.

Index keyword: Trisomy 18 and 13

Support Organisation For Trisomy 13/18 and Related Disorders (SOFT)

7 Orwell Road
Petersfield
Hampshire
GU31 4LQ

Helpline tel: **0121 351 3122**
Admin tel: 01730 261258
Admin fax: 01989 567480
Website: www.SOFT.org.uk

C 🌳 👆 📞 ✏️ 📑 📰 📖

Description: SOFT provides support, assistance and information for families after a pre-natal diagnosis, families with newly diagnosed babies, families caring for surviving children, families experiencing the loss of a child and families wanting another child.

Index keyword: Trisomy 18 and 13

Suzy Lamplugh Trust, The

14 East Sheen Avenue
East Sheen
London
SW14 8AS

Admin tel: 020 8392 1839
Admin fax: 020 8392 1830

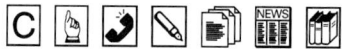

C 👆 📞 ✏️ 📑 📰 📊

Description: As the only organisation in the country specialising in personal safety, the trust aims to create a safer society, providing help and resources for all people. Offers guidance leaflets, posters, manuals, videos, alarms, talks and courses.

Index keyword: General Information

Sympathetic Hearing Scheme

7–11 Armstrong Road
London
W3 7JL

Admin tel: 020 8740 4447
Admin fax: 020 8742 9043

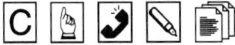

[icons]

Description: Aims to break down communication barriers for deaf and hard of hearing people in public places, by giving them a card they can show to indicate their hearing loss, and by training staff who work with the public to improve their communication skills.

Index keyword: Hearing Problems/Deafness

Tak Tent Cancer Support (SCOTLAND)

Flat 5
30 Shelly Court
Naval Complex
Glasgow
G12 0YN

Helpline tel: **0141 211 1930**
Admin tel: 0141 211 1930
Admin tel: 0141 211 1879
Opening times: 10.00am–3.00pm

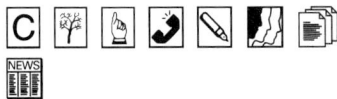

[icons]

Description: Promotes the care of cancer patients, their families, friends and the staff involved professionally in cancer care, by providing information, education, and practical and emotional support.

Index keyword: Cancer

Talking Library for the Indian Blind

21 Hungerford Road
London
N7 9LB

Helpline tel: **020 7609 3590**
Admin tel: 020 7609 3590
Admin fax: 020 7607 4228

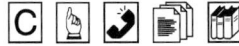

[icons]

Description: Provides books in various Indian languages on standard cassettes.

Index keyword: Blindness/Visual Handicap

Tall Persons Club Great Britain and Ireland

PO Box 163
Stevenage
Herts
S92 9ZY

Admin tel: 07000 825512
Admin fax: 01432 357113

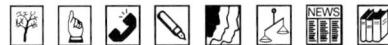

[icons]

Description: Provides information for tall people and promotes their interests.

Index keyword: General Information

Teenage Cancer Trust

Kirkman House
Kirkman Place
54a Tottenham Court Road
London
W1P 9RF
Admin tel: 020 7436 2877
Admin fax: 020 7637 4302

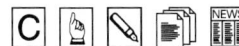

[icons]

Description: Works to establish teenage

cancer units in national health hospitals, for the treatment of adolescents with cancer. These units provide treatment and support, which offer increased recovery chances.

Index keyword: Cancer

Telangiectasia Self-Help Group

39 Sunny Croft
Downley
High Wycombe
Buckinghamshire
HP13 5UQ

Helpline tel: **01494 528047**
Admin tel: 01494 528047
Website: www.tolangiectasia.cwc.net
E-mail: tshg@cwcom.net

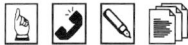

Description: The group was founded in 1985 to maintain a register of sufferers and to put affected families in touch with one another. A newsletter is sent to all members on an occassional basis, informing them of developments in the treatment of this disease.

Index keyword: Telangiectasia

Templegarth Trust

PO Box 6
Louth
Lincolnshire
LN11 8XL

Helpline tel: **0870 7 132584**
Admin fax: 01507 606655

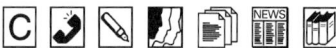

Description: Aims to cultivate health in individuals, families and neighbourhoods and to develop a direct service for health, rather than against disease. Offers, through 'Good Healthkeeping',

information and health counselling; open to family/household membership or casual users, medical referral not required.

Index keyword: Complementary Medicine

Terrence Higgins Trust, The

52–54 Grays Inn Road
London
WC1X 8JU

Helpline tel: **020 7242 1010**
(12.00am–10.00pm)
Admin tel: 020 7831 0330
Admin fax: 020 7242 0121
Website: www.tht.org.uk
E-mail: info@tht.org.uk
Opening times: 9.30am–5.30pm, Mon–Fri

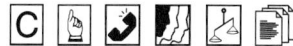

Description: The Terrence Higgins Trust aims to inform, advise and help anyone affected by HIV and AIDS. Our services include counselling, welfare rights, legal and housing advice, library and information service, health promotion work, practical help and a buddy service.

Index keyword: AIDS and HIV

Thalidomide Society

19 Central Avenue
Pinner
Middlesex
HA5 5BT

Helpline tel: **020 8868 5309**
Admin tel: 020 8868 5309
Admin fax: 020 8868 5309
E-mail: info@thalsoc.demon.co.uk
Opening times: 9.00am–5.00pm,
Mon–Thurs

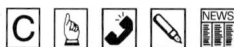

Description: Supports people with thalidomide-related and similar disabilities to overcome their special difficulties. A user-led organisation provides assistance, advice and support to members, professionals and the general public.

Index keyword: Thalidomide

Thyroid Eye Disease Association (TED)

Solstice
Sea Road
Winchelsea Beach
East Sussex
TW36 4LH

Helpline tel: **01797 222338**
Admin tel: 01797 222338
Admin fax: 01797 222338
E-mail: tedassn@eclipse.co.uk
Opening times: 9.00am–5.00pm, Mon–Fri

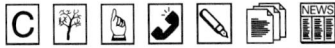

Description: TED provides information, care and support to people affected by thyroid eye disease; has established a network of support groups and telephone helplines throughout the UK; promotes better awareness of the condition among medical profession and public; provides patients with names of hospitals with an awareness of thyroid eye disease; raises money for research.

Index keyword: General Information

Tissue Viability Society

Glanville Centre
Salisbury District Hospital
Salisbury
SP2 8BJ

Helpline tel: **01722 415 069**
(9.00am–3.00pm, Mon & Wed)
Admin tel: 01722 429057
Admin fax: 01722 425263

Website: www.tvs.org.uk
E-mail: tvs@dial.pipex.com
Opening times: 9.00am–5.00pm, Mon – Fri

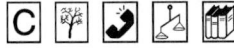

Description: The Society is a unique forum for considering every aspect of the problems associated with tissue viability. Through conferences, publications and study days, members of the various health care disciplines, clinicians and manufacturers in the UK and overseas who share this common interest are brought together.

Index keyword: General Information

Toby Churchill Limited

20 Panton Street
Cambridge
CB2 1HP

Helpline tel: **01223 576117**
Admin tel: 01223 576117
Admin fax: 01223 576118
Website: www.toby-churchill.com
E-mail: sales@toby-churchill.com
Opening times: 9.00am–5.00pm, Mon–Fri

Description: Manufactures, distributes and repairs lightwriters, electronic communication aids for persons with speech difficulties. Lightwriters are keyboard-operated devices with dual displays and optional synthesised speech.

Index keyword: Disability: Equipment

Topaz Postline

BM/TOPAZ
London
WC1N 3XX

Website: www.topazline.org.uk
E-mail: postalcontinuity@hotmail.org.uk

Description: Provides free, friendly, postal counselling, support and befriending for people facing problems they find hard to discuss, or who cannot reach or afford other help. Counselling is open to all and is via letter or tape.

Index keyword: Counselling

Tourette Syndrome (UK) Association, The

The Administration Office
Old Grange House, The Twitten
Southview Road, Crowborough
East Sussex
TN6 1HF

Helpline tel: 01892 669151
Admin tel: 01892 669151
Admin fax: 01892 669151

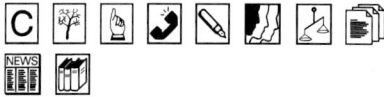

Description: Maintains a register of physicians familiar with the treatment of this disorder. Provides support for people with the disorder and their families. Promotes research and raises funds.

Index keyword: Tourette Syndrome

Traumatic Stress Clinic

73 Charlotte Street
London
W1P 1LB

Helpline tel: 020 7436 900; 020 7530 3666
Admin tel: 020 7530 3666
Admin fax: 020 7530 3677
Website: www.traumatic-stress/tfc.htm
Opening times: 9.00am–5.00pm, Mon–Thurs; 9.00am–4.00pm, Fri

Description: Provides short-term out-patient care for children, families and adults who are survivors of traumatic events.

Index keyword: Stress

Tripscope

Alexandra House
Albany Road
Brentford
Middlesex
TW8 0NE

Admin tel: 020 8580 7021
Admin fax: 020 8580 7022

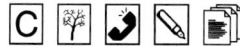

Description: Tripscope is a nationwide travel and transport information and advice service for disabled and elderly people.

Index keyword: Disability: General Information

Triumph Over Phobia (Top UK)

PO Box 1831
Bath
BA2 4YW

Admin tel: 01225 330353
Admin fax: 01225 469212
E-mail: triumphoverphobia@compuserve

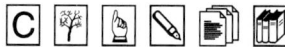

Description: Their main aim is to help people suffering from phobia and obsessive compulsive disorder (OCD) to become ex-sufferers, by learning self-management of their phobia or OCD in structured self-help groups. Contact head office for a list of current groups.

Index keyword: Phobias

Trust for the Study of Adolescence

23 New Road
Brighton
BN1 1WZ

Helpline tel: **01273 693311**
Admin tel: 01273 693311
Admin fax: 01273 679907
Website: www.tsa.uk.com
E-mail: info@tsa.uk.com
Opening times: 9.00am–5.00pm, Mon–Fri

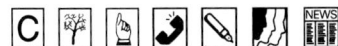

[C] [pencil] [book]

Description: Aims to foster and stimulate research on adolescent development; to address social issues and their impact on young people; to disseminate information on adolescence to parents, to professionals and to the public; to represent the needs of young people, especially those suffering disadvantage or disability.

Index keyword: General Information

Turning Point

New Loom House
101 Backchurch Lane
London
E1 1LU

Helpline tel: **020 7702 2300**
Admin tel: 020 7702 2300
Admin fax: 020 7702 1456
Website: www.turning-point.co.uk
E-mail: tpmail@turningpoint.co.uk
Opening times: 9.00am–5.00pm, Mon–Fri

[C] [tree] [hand] [phone] [pencil] [foot] [NEWS]

Description: Turning point is the largest national charity helping people with drug and alcohol problems, mental health problems and learning disabilities.

Index keyword: Drug Addiction/Side Effects

Twins And Multiple Births Association (TAMBA)

Harnott House
309 Chester Road
Little Sutton
Ellesmere Port
CH66 1QQ

Helpline tel: **01732 868000**
(7.00pm–11.00pm, weekdays;
10.00am–11.00pm, weekends)
Admin tel: 0870 1214000
Admin fax: 0870 1214001
Website: www.surrey.org.uk/tamba
Opening times: 7.00pm–11.00pm, Mon–Fri
10.00am–11.00pm, weekends

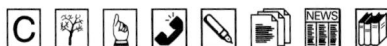

[C] [tree] [hand] [phone] [pencil] [papers] [NEWS] [book]

Description: Supports families with twins, triplets or more children, individually and through local twins clubs and specialist support groups. Promotes public and professional awareness of their needs. TAMBA's other support groups are: one parent families; bereavement; infertility; adopted multiples; and special needs, adults and supertwins.

Index keyword: Children: General Information

Typetalk

John Wood House
Glacier Building
Harrington Road
Brunswick Business Park
Liverpool
L3 4DF

Helpline tel: **0800 500888**
Admin tel: 0151 709 9494
Admin fax: 0151 709 8119
E-mail: helpline@rnib-typetalk.org.uk
Opening times: 24 hours

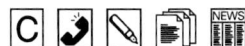

[C] [phone] [pencil] [papers] [NEWS]

Description: Typetalk is the national telephone relay service run by the RNID and funded by BT, which enables deaf/speech-impaired people to communicate with hearing people anywhere in the world over the telephone network. The Text Users' Rebate Scheme offers substantial help with phone bills to people who are deaf/speech-impaired.

Index keyword: Hearing Problems/ Deafness

U

UK Council for Psychotherapy

167–169 Great Portland Street
London
W1N 5FB

Admin tel: 020 7436 3002
Admin fax: 020 7436 3013
Website: www.psychotherapy.org.uk
E-mail: ukcp@psychotherapy.org.uk

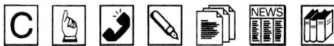

Description: Promotes and maintains the profession of psychotherapy and high standards of practice, as the umbrella body for all approaches to psychotherapy practised in the UK. Holds the National Register of Psychotherapists and provides the public with lists of registered practitioners working in their area.

Index keyword: Psychotherapy

UK Homoeopathic Medical Association

6 Livingstone Road
Gravesend
Kent
DA12 5DZ

Helpline tel: **01474 560336**
Admin tel: 01474 560336
Admin fax: 01474 327431
Website: www,the-hma.org.uk
E-mail: info@the-hma.org

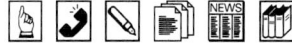

Description: The UKHMA is an association of qualified professional homoeopaths. Members are bound by a strict code of ethics and obliged to carry professional indemnity insurance, so that the public may seek treatment with absolute confidence.

Index keyword: Complementary Medicine

UK Thalassaemia Society

19 The Broadway
Southgate Circus
London
N14 6PH

Helpline tel: **020 8882 0011**
Admin fax: 020 8882 8618
Website: www.ukts.org.uk
E-mail: office@ukts.org.uk

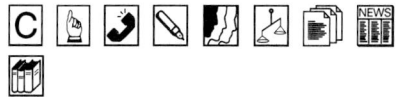

Description: Aims to relieve the suffering caused by thalassaemia; to promote, fund and co-ordinate research in connection with thalassaemia; to raise awareness of the problems it causes; to offer counselling to sufferers and their carers; and to bring together parents, families and well-wishers to exchange ideas and information.

Index keyword: Sickle Cell/Thalassaemia

UKHCA

4 Banstead Road
Carshalton Beeches
Surrey
SM5 3NW

Helpline tel: **020 8288 1555**
Admin tel: 020 8288 1551
Admin fax: 020 8288 1550
Website: www.ukhca.co.uk
E-mail: enquiries@ukhca.demon.co.uk

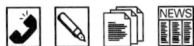

Description: The UKHCA is the national representative association for home care organisations which provide care, including nursing care, to people in their own homes. Its primary aim is to identify and promote the highest standards of home care.

Index keyword: General Information

Ulster Cancer Foundation

40–42 Eglantine Avenue
Belfast
BT9 6DX

Helpline tel: **0800 7833339**
Admin tel: 02890 663281
Admin fax: 02890 660081
Opening times: 9.00am–5.00pm,Mon–Fri

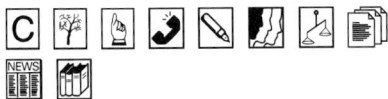

Description: Helps people who are suffering from the effects of cancer, either themselves or in their family. Has a comprehensive range of services: experienced cancer counselling; patient to patient home and hospital visits; support groups; telephone helpline; patient advice centre, with advice on medical supplies, speech aids, prostheses and specialist clothing.

Index keyword: Cancer

United Kingdom Advocacy Network

14–18 West Bar Green
Sheffield
S1 2DA

Helpline tel: **0114 272 8171**
Admin tel: 0114 272 8171
Admin fax: 0114 272 8171
E-mail: ukcan@cam-online.org.uk
Opening times: 9.00am–5.00pm, Mon–Fri

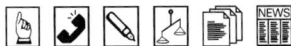

Description: Provides advice, information and training on mental health service user empowerment, National Federation of Patients' Councils, user forums and advocacy groups.

Index keyword: Mental Health/Illness

'Unwind' (Pain and Stress Management)

Melrose
3 Alderlea Close
Gilesgate
Durham
DH1 1DS

Helpline tel: **0191 384 2056**
Admin tel: 0191 384 2056
Admin fax: 0191 384 2056
Opening times: publications by mail *only*

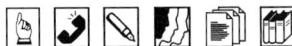

Description: Aims to bring hope and direction to sufferers of pain and stress, to provide structured self-help programmes, to enable sufferers to take control of their own particular situation.

Index keyword: Stress

V

Values Into Action

Oxford House
Derbyshire Street
London
E2 6HG

Admin tel: 020 7729 5436
Admin fax: 020 7729 7797

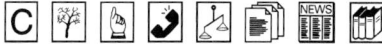

Description: Values Into Action is a campaigning organisation committed to achieving laws, services and public attitudes which will allow people with learning disabilities to become valued citizens.

Index keyword: Mental Health/Illness

VBAC Information and Support

8 Wren Way
Farnborough
Hampshire
GU14 8SZ

Helpline tel: 01252 677658
Admin tel: 01252 677658
E-mail: linda.VBAC@tesco.net

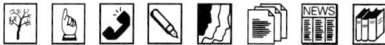

Description: VBAC was set up to help women who wish to avoid unnecessary surgery for the birth of their babies.

Index keyword: Pregnancy and Childbirth

Victim Support

National Office
Cranmer House
39 Brixton Road
London
SW9 6DZ

Helpline tel: 0845 30 30 9000 (Mon–Fri, 9.00am–9.00pm; Sat–Sun, 9.00am–7.00pm)
Admin tel: 020 7735 9166
Admin fax: 020 7582 5712
Opening times: 9.00am–5.30pm, Mon–Fri

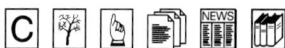

Description: This is a national charity working for victims of crime. Staff and trained volunteers in local schemes and crown court witness services provide emotional support, practical help and information to victims and witnesses of crime. Works to increase understanding and awareness of effects of crime and to gain better recognition of victims' rights.

Index keyword: General Information

Voluntary Transcribers' Group

8 Segbourne Road
Rubery
Birmingham
B45 9SX

Helpline tel: 0121 453 4268
Admin tel: 0121 453 4268
Admin fax: 0870 1228613
Website:
hwtp://ds.dial.pipex.com/batchelor
E-mail: batchelor@dial.pipex.com
Opening times: All day

Description: Provides a transcription service of print into braille.

Index keyword: Blindness/Visual Handicap

W

Wales Council for The Blind

3rd Floor
Shand House
20 Newport Road
Cardiff
CF24 0DB

Helpline tel: **01222 473954**
Admin tel: 01222 473954
Admin fax: 029 2004 33920
Website: www.wcbnet.freeserve.co.uk
E-mail: staff@wcbnet.freeserve.co.uk
Opening times: 9.00am–5.00pm, Mon–Fri

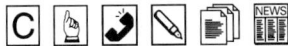

Description: Aims to enable and empower visually impaired people, by monitoring services in Wales, promoting services where they do not exist, encouraging improvement in standards in services, supporting voluntary efforts and co-ordinating statutory and voluntary efforts.

Index keyword: Blindness/Visual Handicap

Well Being

27 Sussex Place
Regents Park
London
NW1 4SP

Helpline tel: **020 7262 5337**
Admin tel: 020 7262 5337
Admin fax: 020 7724 7725
Website: www.wellbeing.demon.co.uk
E-mail: wb239281@aol.com
Opening times: Mon–Fri

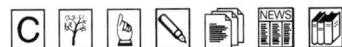

Description: Well Being, the health research charity for women and babies, is the research arm of The Royal College of Obstetricians and Gynaecologists. They fund research into all matters of women's health, and educate and inform women on related matters. Provides leaflets.

Index keyword: Women's Health

Wellbeing Initiative

Clydeway Centre
45 Finnieston Street
Glasgow
G3 8JU

Helpline tel: **0141 248 1899**
Admin tel: 0141 248 1899
Admin fax: 0141 248 1899
E-mail: wellbeing@hotmail.com
Opening times: 9.00am–5.00pm,
Mon–Thurs; 9.00am–4.00pm, Fri

Description: Wellbeing is a health and disability information service, with an up-to-date store of information on all aspects of health and disability, specialising in self-help groups. Wellbeing is also a training centre for people with physical disabilities, providing training for level I-II Scotvec (SVQ) in Business Administration.

Index keyword: Disability: General Information

Wessex Cancer Trust Marc's Line (Melanoma And Related Cancers of the Skin)

Dermatology Treatment Centre
Level 3, Salisbury District Hospital
Salisbury
Wiltshire
SP2 8BJ

Helpline tel: **01722 415071**
Admin tel: 01722 415071
Admin fax: 01722 415071

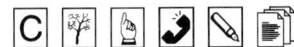

Description: Marc's Line is a resource centre and telephone advice line. It seeks to be of value to patients and their families, health professionals, teachers and others involved in education about skin cancer or its prevention. Marc's Line is funded by Wessex Cancer Trust and affiliated to the Dermatology Department of Salisbury District Hospital.

Index keyboard: Cancer

West Syndrome Support Group

8 Waddon Close
Croydon
CR0 4JT

Helpline tel: **020 8680 8449**
Opening times: 9.00am–5.00pm, Mon–Fri

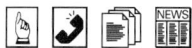

Description: The group aims to raise awareness, provide information and link affected families.

Index keyword: West Syndrome

Why me?

6 Thorney Close
Fareham
Hampshire
PO14 3AF

Helpline tel: **01329 312997**
Admin tel: 01329 312997

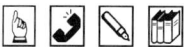

Description: Provides help and guidance to sufferers from acute anxiety disorder, agoraphobia and panic attacks, and to their families and friends.

Index keyword: Anxiety

Williams Syndrome Foundation Limited

161 High Street
Tonbridge
Kent
TN9 1BX

Helpline tel: **01732 365152**
Admin fax: 01732 360178
Website: www.williams-syndrome.org.uk

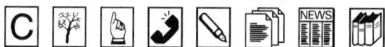

Description: The foundation was formed in 1980 for the twin purposes of research and of giving help and support to families with affected children. It incorporates Williams syndrome and infantile hypercalcaemia. Offers an information and advisory service; pays for group holiday weeks for unaccompanied adults and for families.

Index keyword: General Information

Winter Warmth Line

Help The Aged
St James's Walk
Clerkenwell Green
London
EC1R 0BE

Helpline tel: **0800 289404**
Admin tel: 020 7253 0253
Admin fax: 020 7251 0747
Website: www.helptheaged

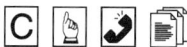

Description: Help The Aged runs the Winter Warmth Line for six months each year (October–March), as part of the annual Keep Warm Keep Well campaign. Telephone advice is given on how to keep yourself and your home warm, and on other winter issues.

Index keyword: Elderly: General Information

Wireless for the Bedridden Society (Inc), The

159a High Street
Hornchurch
Essex
RM11 3YB

Helpline tel: **0800 0182 137**
Admin tel: 01708 621101
Admin fax: 01708 620816
Opening times: 8.45am–4.30pm, Mon–Fri

Description: Provides radio and television sets to housebound, disabled and elderly people who are unable to afford a set for themselves.

Index keyword: Disability: Equipment

Women Of the Beaumont Society (WOBS)

27 Old Gloucester Street
London
WC1N 3XX

Helpline tel: **01223 441246**
Admin tel: 01223 441246
Website: www.members.aol.com/wobsuk
E-mail: wobsuk@aol.com
Opening times: 10.00am–10.00pm, Mon–Fri

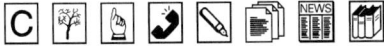

Description: Provides support for anyone who is closely connected to a person who cross-dresses. Networks with related organisations and professionals to maintain, update and extend its service.

Index keyword: Gays/Lesbians

Women's Alcohol Centre

66a Drayton Park
London
N5 1ND

Helpline tel: **020 7226 4581**
Admin fax: 020 7354 8134

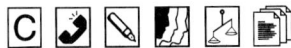

Description: The Centre offers an individual counselling service and group work programme for women who are concerned about their drinking. Offers residential places to women who are homeless or feel that a period of time away from their home environment would be beneficial. Aims to help women look at the problems around their drinking and find alternative ways of handling them.

Index keyword: Alcohol Problems

Women's Health

52 Featherstone Street
London
EC1Y 8RT

Helpline tel: **020 7251 6580**
Admin tel: 020 7251 6333
Admin fax: 020 7608 0928
Website:
www.womenshealthlondon.org.uk
Opening times: 10.00am–4.00pm,
Mon–Wed; 10.00am–1.00pm, Thurs, Fri

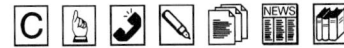

Description: Provides unbiased information on a wide range of topics concerning women's health issues, helping women to make informed choices. Has a library open to the public.

Index keyword: Women's Health

Women's Nutritional Advisory Service

PO Box 268
Lewes
East Sussex
BN7 2QN

Admin tel: 01273 487366
Admin fax: 01273 487576
E-mail: wnas@wnas.org.uk

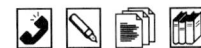

Description: Tailor-made programmes for PMS, menopause, IBS, sugar craving, preconceptual care; fatigue dietary and nutritional advice. Clinics and telephone consultation service.

Index keyword: Nutrition/Diet

Womens Nationwide Cancer Control Campaign (WNCCC)

Suna House
128–130 Curtain Road
London
EC2A 3AQ

Admin tel: 020 7729 4688; 020 7729 1735
Admin fax: 020 7613 0771
Website: www.wncc.org.uk
E-mail: wncc@admin.co.uk
Opening times: 9.00am–5.00pm, Mon–Fri

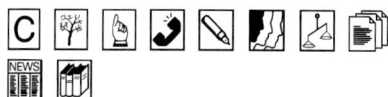

Description: The WNCCC supports and encourages the provision of facilities for the early diagnosis of cancer, primarily breast, cervical and ovarian. It produces a wide range of publications and some videos, gives health talks, for homeless women and women who fall through the statutory net.

Index keyword: Cancer

Working With Men

320 Commercial Way
London
SE15 1QN

Admin tel: 020 7732 9409
Admin fax: 020 7732 9409

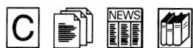

Description: WWM supports the development of work through resources, publications, training, consultancy and advice to professional – very active in men's health and young men's education.

Index keyword: Men's Health

WPF Counselling

23 Kensington Square
London
W8 5HN

Helpline tel: **020 7937 6956**
Admin tel: 020 7361 4800
Admin fax: 020 7361 4808
Website: www.wpf.org.uk/counsken.html
E-mail: counselling@wpf.org.uk
Opening times: 8.00am–8.00pm, Mon–Fri

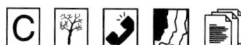

Description: Offers counselling for individuals (including young people and the physically ill) and group therapy. The theoretic orientation is psychodynamic. WPF is a member of BAC and UKCP. There is a sliding scale of fees. Training for counsellors and psychotherapists is provided by WPF Kensington (Institute of Psychotherapy and Counselling).

Index keyword: Psychotherapy

Write Away

29 Crawford Street
London
W1H 1PL

Helpline tel: **020 7724 0878**
Admin tel: 020 7724 0878
Admin fax: 020 7724 0878

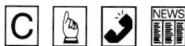

Description: Write Away is a penfriend club for children with special needs (aged 8–18) and their brothers and sisters.

Index keyword: Disability: Children

Yoga for Health Foundation

Ickwell Bury
Biggleswade
SG18 9EF

Admin tel: 01767 627271
Admin fax: 01767 627445
Opening times: Mon–Fri

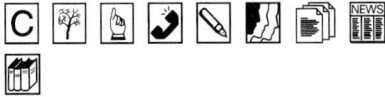

C ☘ 👆 ☎ ✏ 🦵 📑 📰 📖

Description: This is a residential yoga centre, specialising in working with people with disability and chronic ill health.

Index keyword: Complementary Medicine

You and Yours

BBC Broadcasting House
Room 6122
BBC Radio 4
BBC Broadcasting House
London
W1A 1AA

Helpline tel: **020 7765 2383**
Admin tel: 020 7765 2383
Admin fax: 020 7765 5157
Website: www.bbc.co.uk
E-mail: youandyours@bbc.co.uk

Description: Consumer and investigative programme which also covers disabilities.

Young Minds

102–108 Clerkenwell Road
London
EC1M 5SA

Helpline tel: **0800 018 2138**
Admin tel: 020 7336 8445
Admin fax: 020 7336 8446
Website: www.youngminds.org.uk
E-mail: enquiries@youngminds.org.uk
Opening times: 10.00am–1.00pm, Mon & Fri; 1.00pm–4.00pm, Tues–Thurs

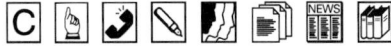

C 👆 ☎ ✏ 🦵 📑 📰 📖

Description: Young Minds exists to increase awareness of the mental health needs of young people and their families; to offer an information and advice line for any adult concerned about the emotional welfare of a young person.

Index keyword: Mental Health/Illness

Young People's Consultation Service

Tavistock Clinic
120 Belsize Lane
London
NW3 5BA

Helpline tel: **020 7447 3787**
Admin tel: 020 7435 7111
Opening times: 9.00am–5.00pm, Mon–Fri

🦵

Description: Offers free and confidential counselling within the NHS to anyone between the ages of 16 and 30 who has a personal or emotional problem.

Index keyword: Counselling

Zito Trust, The

PO Box 265
London
WC2H 9JD

Helpline tel: **01497 820011**
Admin tel: 01497 820011
Admin fax: 01497 820011
Opening times: Mon–Fri

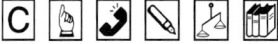

Description: The Zito Trust is a registered charity, established to work for improvements in the provision of community care for the severely mentally ill, by providing a network of support for families and professional carers who find themselves at risk or bereaved, owing to failure in the provision of care.

Index keyword: Mental Health/Illness

Index

A

Alzheimer's Disease

Alzheimer Scotland (Action on Dementia)   11
Alzheimer's Disease Society   12
Alzheimer's Disease Society (Northern Ireland)   12

Amputees

British Limbless Ex Servicemen's Association (BLESMA)   36
Limbless Association   114

Angelman Syndrome

Angelman Syndrome Support Group   13

Ankylosing Spondylitis

National Ankylosing Spondylitis Society   131

Anxiety

Why Me?   204

Arthritis/Rheumatic Disorders

Arthritic Association   15
Arthritis Care   15
Children's Chronic Arthritis Association   53
Horder Centre for Arthritis, The   96

Asthma

Action Asthma Patient service   3
Midlands Asthma and Allergy Research Association   126
National Asthma Campaign   135

Autism

International Autistic Research Organisation, The (Autism Research Limited)   101
National Autistic Society, The   135
Scottish Society for Autism   182
Society for the Autisitically Handicapped (SFTAH)   189

B

Beckwith Wiedemann Syndrome

Beckwith Wiedemann Support Group   23

Bereavement

Action for Victims of Medical Accidents   4
Child Bereavement Trust, The   51
Child Death Helpline   51
Compassionate Friends, The   56
Cruse Bereavement Care (Northern Ireland)   63
Faithfully Yours   80
London Bereavement Network   115
Scottish Cot Death Trust   180
Stillbirth And Neonatal Death Society (SANDS)   193
Sudden Death Support Association   194

Blindness/Visual Handicapped

ADA Reading Service for the Blind   6
British Council for Prevention of Blindness   32
British Retinitis Pigmentosa Society   39
British Wireless for the Blind fund   42
Calibre   43
Clearvision Project   55
Electronic Aids for the Blind   76
Guide Dogs for the Blind Association   88
Guide Dogs for the Blind Association, The   88
In Touch Publishing   98
Listening Books   114
Living Paintings Trust, The   114
National Federation of the Blind   139
National Music for the Blind   141
Partially Sighted Society   156
Playback Recording Service for the Blind   159
RNIB (Northern Ireland)   172
RNIB Talking book Service   172
RNIB Transcription Centre Northwest   173
Royal National Institute for the Blind   176
Seeability   183
Sight Savers International   187
Talking Library for the Indian Blind   195
Voluntary Transcribers' Group   202
Wales Council for the Blind   202

Bone Marrow

Anthony Nolan Bone Marrow Trust, The   13

Bowel

Irritable Bowel Syndrome Network (IBS Network)   104

Brain Injuries

Association for Brain Damaged Children and Young Adults, The   16

Brittle Bones Society

Brittle Bone Society   43

C

Cancer

Action against Breast Cancer   3

Care Scheme/Holidays

Carers

C

Cerebral Palsy

Childcare

Children

Chiropractic

Cleft Lip/Palate

Colitis

Complementary Medicine

Cornelia De Lange Syndrome

Cosmetic Surgery

Cot Death

Counselling

Couples Counselling

Cri Du Chat Syndrome

Crohn's Disease

Cushing Syndrome

Cystic Fibrosis

Cystitis

D

Death and Bereavement

Dental Health

Depression

DES Exposure

Diabetes

Digestive Problems

Disability

D

Disfigurement

Divorce/Separation

Down's Syndrome

Drug Addiction/Side Effects

Dyslexia

Dystonia

E

Eating Disorders

Eclampsia

F

Farby's Disease

Fabry Disease Research Fund and Support Group   79

Families

Special Families Trust   191

Family Planing

Family Planning Association Scotland   81
Family Planning Association Wales   82
Fertility UK   83
International Planned Parenthood Federation   102

Family Support and Welfare

Family Action Information and Resource (FAIR)   80
Family Service Units   82
Family Welfare Association   82
Home-Start UK   95
National Council for One Parent Families   137

Feet

Society of Chiropodists and Podiatrists   190

First Aid

St John Ambulance   192

Food

Food Commission, The   84

G

Gambling

Gamcare   85
Parents of Young Gamblers   156

Gardening

Gardening for the Disabled   86
Royal Gardeners Orphan Fund, The   175
Society for Horticultural Therapy   189

Gaucher's Disease

Gauchers Association   86

Gays/Lesbian

Campaign for Homosexual Equality   44
Lesbian and Gay Bereavement Project   111
Lesbian and Gay Christian Movement   112
Lesbian and Gay Employment Rights   112
Lesbian Line   112
London Lesbian and Gay Switchboard   116
Parents' Friend   156
Project for Advice, Counselling and Education (PACE)   163
Women Of the Beaumont Society (WOBS)   205

General Health

Appropriate Health Resources and Technologies Action Group (AHRTAG)   14
Healthline Health Information Service   92
Healthwise Helpline   92
Independent Healthcare Association   99
Keep Fit Association   107
London Chinese Health Resource Centre   116
NHS Confederation   147
NHS Direct   147
NHS Helpline   147
Public Health Alliance, The   165
Scottish Association of Health Councils   180
Self Help Team, The   183

General Information

Able Community Care   1
Acorns Childrens Hospice   2
Action 19 Plus   2
Action for Dysphasic Adults (ADA)   3
Action on Elder Abuse   4
Age Concern Cymru   7
Age Concern England   8
Age Concern Scotland   8
Air Transport Users Council   8
Amnesty International UK   12
Association for Glycogen Storage Disease, The (UK)   17
Association of Charity Officers, The   18
Association of Parents of Vaccine Damaged Children   19
Association to aid the Sexual and Personal Relationships of People with a Disability, The (SPOD)   20
Ataxia   20
Attia Research Trust into ALD   21
Banstead Mobility Centre   22
Beaumont Society, The   23
Benefit Enquiry Line for People with Disabilities   23
Birmingham Tapes for the Handicapped Association   24
Blue Cross   25
Bourne Trust, The   26
Bretforton Academy, The   27

G

Prevention of Professional Abuse Network
(POPAN)   162
Prison Reform Trust   163
Professional Classes Aid Council   163
Purine Metabolic Patients Association
(PUMPA)   165
Queen Elizabeth's Foundation for Disabled
People   165
Radionic   166
RCN Work Injured Nurses Group   167
Reflex Anoxic Seizure Information and
Support Group   169
Restricted Growth Association   171
RICA   171
Richard Wilson Accessible Transport Services
171
RNIB Multiple Disability Services   172
Road Peace   173
Royal Agricultural Benevolent Institution   173
Royal Association for Disability And
Rehabilitation (RADAR)   174
Salvation Army   177
Salvation Army   178
Salvation Army Family Tracing Service, The
178
Senior Line   183
Sequal Trust, The   184
Seriously Ill for Medical Research (SIMR)   184
Sesame Institute UK   185
SHARE Community Ltd   185
Shipwreck Mariners' Society   186
Skill (National Bureau for Students with
Disabilities)   188
Snowdon Award Scheme   188
Society for Mucopolysaccharide Diseases, The
189
SOS Talisman   191
St Vincent de Paul Society (England and
Wales)   192
Streetwise Youth   193
Sturge-Weber Foundation (UK)   193
Suzy Lamplugh Trust, The   194
Tall Persons Club Great Britain and
Ireland   195
Thyroid Eye Disease Association (TED)   197
Tissue Viability Society   197
Tripscope   198
Trust for the Study of Adolescence   199
Twins and Multiple Births Association
(TAMBA)   199
UKHCA   200
Victim Support   202
Wellbeing Initiative   203
Williams syndrome Foundation Limited   204
Winter Warmth Line   204

Genetics

Genetic Interest Group   86

Gifted Children

Gifted Children's Information Centre   87

Growth Problems

Child Growth Foundation   52

Guillain–Barré Syndrome

Guillain–Barré Syndrome Support Group of
the United Kingdom   89

H

Haemochromatosis

Haemochromatosis Society   89

Haemophilia

Haemophilia Society, The   90
Newcastle Haemophilia Comprehensive Care
Centre   146

Hair

Hairline International Alopecia Patients'
Society (The)   90

Head Injury

Children's Head Injury Trust   53
Headway: Brain Injury Association   91

Hearing Problems/Deafness

Beethoven Fund for Deaf Children, The   23
Breakthrough (Deaf/Hearing Integration)   26
British Deaf Association Health Promotion
Unit   32
British Tinnitus Association   42
Catholic Deaf Association   48
Council for the Advancement of
Communication with Deaf People   61
Deaf Broadcasting Council   65
FYD (Friends for Young Deaf People)   85
Hearing Dogs for the Deaf   92
Hearing Research Trust   92
Link Centre for Deafened People   114
National Deaf Childrens' Society   137
National Deafblind League   138
Paget Gorman Society, The   153
RNID Tinnitus Helpline   173
Royal Association in Aid of Deaf People   174
Royal National Institute for Deaf People (Head
Office)   175
Royal National Institute for Death People
(Northern Ireland)   175

I

K

L

L

Learning Disabilities

British Institute of Learning Disabilities   36
Mencap (Royal Society for Mentally
    Handicapped Children and Adults)   123
Mencap in Northern Ireland   123

Lefthanded

Anything Left-Handed Limited   14
Left-Handed Company   110

Leprosy

LEPRA (The British Leprosy Relief
    Association)   111

Leukaemia

Leukaemia Care Society, The   113
Leukaemia Research Fund   113

Liver Disease

British Liver Trust   37
Children's Liver Disease Foundation   54

Lung Disease

British Lung Foundation (Breathe Easy Club)
    37

Lupus Erythematosus

Lupus UK   117

Lymphoedema

Lymphoedema Support Network   117

M

Marfan Syndrome

Marfan Association UK   118

Marriage

Marriage Care   119
RELATE   170

ME (Myalgic Encephalomyelitis)

Action for ME   3
ME Association   121
National ME Centre   141

Mediation

Mediation UK   121

Meningitis

Meningitis Research Foundation   124
National Meningitis Trust   141

Men's Health

Male Advice Line and Enquiries (MALE)   118
Men's Health Matters   123
Working With Men   206

Mental Health/Illness

Arbours Association Limited   14
Association for Residential Care   18
Camphill Village Trust   44
Caring and Sharing Trust   47
Cottage And Rural Enterprises Limited
    (CARE)   60
Dementia Services Development Centre   66
Ex-Services Mental Welfare Society   78
Guideposts Trust Limited   89
L'Arche   109
Matthew Trust, The   121
Mencap in Northern Ireland   123
Mental After Care Association (MACA)   124
Mental Health Act Commission   124
Mental Health Foundation Scotland   124
Mental Health Foundation, The   125
Mental Health Media   125
Mind (The Mental Health Charity)   126
NAPSAC   130
National Federation of Gateway Clubs   139
Praxis Mental Health   161
Psychiatric Rehabilitation Association (PRA)   164
Rathbone CI   166
Reading Cygnets Swimming Club for the
    Mentally Handicapped   168
RESCARE (The National Society for Mentally
    Handicapped People in Residential Care)   171
Richmond Fellowship   172
Royal College of Psychiatrists   175
Scottish Association for Mental Health   179
United Kingdom Advocacy Network   201
Values into Action   201
Young Minds   207
Zito Trust, The   208

Migraine

British Migraine Association   37
Migraine Trust, The   126

Motor Neurone Diseases

Motor Neurone Disease Association   128

THE HEALTH ADDRESS BOOK 2000–2001: A Directory of Health Support Groups

P

Phenylketonuria

NSPKU   150

Phobias

Anxiety and Phobia Network   14
No Panic   148
Phobics Society, The   158
Triumph Over Phobia (Top UK)   198

Plastic Surgery

British Association of Aesthetic Plastic
    Surgeons   29

Polio

British Polio Fellowship   38
Northern Ireland Polio Fellowship   149

Polyartertis

Polyartertis Contact List   159

Prader-Willi Syndrome

Prader-Willi Syndrome Association (UK)   161

Pregnancy and Childbirth

Action on Pre-Eclampsia (APEC)   5
Anti-Natal Results and Choices (ARC)   13
Association for Improvements in the Maternity
    Services (AIMS)   18
Association of Radical Midwives   20
Birth Centre Limited, The   24
Birth Defects Foundation   25
British Pregnancy Advisory Services   38
Caroline Flint Midwifery Services   47
Centre for Pregnancy Nutrition   49
Childlessness Overcome through Surrogacy   52
Disabled Parents Network   71
Foresight (The Association for the Promotion
    of Pre-Conceptual Care)   84
Leeds Antenatal Screening Service   110
Life Pregnancy Care Centre   113
Maternity Alliance, The   120
Meet-A-Mum-Association   122
Miscarriage Association, The   127
National Childbirth Trust   136
Parentability (Disabled Parents Network)   155
Pre-Eclampsia Society   161
Society for the Protection of Unborn Children
    189
VBAC Information and Support   202

Premenstrual Syndrome

National Association For premenstrual
    Syndrome (NAPS)   132

PMS Help   159
Premenstrual society   162

Prostate

Prostate Association   163

Psychology

British Psychological Society   39

Psychotherapy

Association for Humanistic Psychology   17
British Association of Psychotherapists, The
    30
Child Psychotherapists Trust, The   52
Guild of Psychotherapists, The   89
London Centre for Psychotherapists and
    psychotherapists   115
National Register of Hypnotherapy and
    Psychotherapists   143
Philadelphia Association   158
Psychotherapy Centre, The   165
UK Council for Psychotherapy   200
WPF Counselling   206

R

Rape/Battered Women

Incestuous Relationship and Rape   99
London Rape Crisis Centre   116

Raynauds Disease

Raynaud's and Scleroderma Association   167

Research

Action Research   5

Reyes' Syndrome

National Reye's Syndrome Foundation of the
    UK   143

S

Schizophrenia

Forresters (National Schizophrenia Fellowship)
    84
Making Space   117
National Schizophrenia Fellowship (NSF)   144

T

V

Thalidomide

Thelidomide Society   196

Thyroid

British Thyroid Foundation   42

Tourette Syndrome

Tourette syndrome (UK) Association, The   198

Travel

Medical Advisory Services for Travellers
Abroad (MASTA)   122

Trisomy 18 and 13

Support Organisations For Trisomy 13 /18 and
Related Disorders (SOFT)   194
Support Organisation For Trisomy (UK)
(SOFT)   194

V

Victims

Criminal Injuries Compensation Authority   62

Volunteers

Community Service Volunteers (CSV)   56
National Association of Councils for Voluntary
Service   134
REACH   168

W

West Syndrome

West Syndrome Support Group   204

Women's Health

Breast Care Campaign   27
Kingston Women's Centre   108
London Black Women's Register   115
Scottish Women's Aid   182
Women's Health   205

Entry form

Please provide a contact name in case we need to contact you about your entry

Mr/Mrs/Miss/Ms ——————————————— Tel: ———————————

Name of organisation: ———————————————————————

Address of organisation: ——————————————————————

——————————————————————

Helpline Telephone: ————————————————
(please indicate opening times if not normal office hours) ———————————

Admin Telephone: ————————— Fax: ————————————

General (please circle)

Are you a charity   YES/NO

Do you have branches/local groups   YES/NO

Do you use volunteers in your work   YES/NO

Advice/support (please tick)

❏   Telephone advice   ❏   Counselling

❏   Written advice   ❏   Advocacy

Publications (please tick)

❏   Information leaflets   ❏   Books/other publications (please describe)

❏   Newsletter   ———————————————

Aims & other activities (50 words max.)

❏   **Please tick here if you would like to receive further information about the Patients Association.**

Please return to The Patients Association, 8 Guilford Street, London WC1N 1DT